Emerging Issues in Family and Individual Resilience

Series Editors
Amanda W. Harrist, Oklahoma State University
Stillwater, OK, USA

Each year the Oklahoma State University's Center for Family Resilience holds a conference where distinguished and rising scholars from diverse disciplines discuss cutting-edge work and foster the community of educators and researchers in the field of family resilience. Presenting research-based knowledge from a range of academic disciplines such as family studies, human development, psychology, sociology, social work, education, law, and medicine, the series facilitates the development of evidence-based resilience practices, programs, and policies for those working with families at risk.

Julie M. Koch • Erica E. Townsend-Bell
Randolph D. Hubach
Editors

Identity as Resilience in Minoritized Communities

Strengths-Based Approaches to Research and Practice

Springer

Editors
Julie M. Koch
University of Iowa
Iowa City, IA, USA

Erica E. Townsend-Bell
Oklahoma State University
Stillwater, OK, USA

Randolph D. Hubach
Purdue University
West Lafayette, IN, USA

ISSN 2366-6072 ISSN 2366-6080 (electronic)
Emerging Issues in Family and Individual Resilience
ISBN 978-3-031-38976-4 ISBN 978-3-031-38977-1 (eBook)
https://doi.org/10.1007/978-3-031-38977-1

This Springer imprint is published by the registered company Springer Nature Switzerland AG
The registered company address is: Gewerbestrasse 11, 6330 Cham, Switzerland

Paper in this product is recyclable.

We dedicate this book to those who know that marginality is neither the beginning nor the end. Fight on.

Preface

We are excited to introduce this volume, *Identity as Resilience in Minoritized Communities: Strengths-Based Approaches to Understanding Minoritized Communities*, to readers.[1] The chapters here reflect work presented by nationally recognized scholars at the 2021 and 2022 Chautauqua Conferences on Family Resilience. The 2021 conference, "Resilience of LGBTQ+ Families: Pride and Celebration," focused on family resilience and affirmative work with families with members with lesbian, gay, bisexual, transgender, queer, or gender-expansive identities. The 2022 conference, "Identity as Resilience: Strengths Based Approaches to Development among Youth, Family, and Community," continued the theme of identity and community, specifically related to race and ethnicity, as a source of strength and resilience.

About the Chautauqua Conference and This Series

Chautauqua is an Iroquois word meaning something similar to "bag tied in the middle" or "two moccasins tied together." Among other things, this word described a lake located in New York where the Iroquois nation was located. The word was then taken and used by White settlers to refer to a series of assemblies for dialogue and education in the late nineteenth and early twentieth centuries. The tradition continues with the annual Chautauqua Conference on Family Resilience at Oklahoma State University, which began in 2008 in hopes of continuing the mission of education that was not limited to the "ivory tower," but shared with and co-created with the people, a clear match with the University's land grant mission. In this way, Chautauqua history, like so much of American history, is complicated and carries roots of inequality and injustice bound up with its loftier democratic goals. The goal

[1] We use the terms minoritized and marginalized as interchangeable synonyms. Both concepts highlight the point that minority status is a result of social and political processes rather than a neutral demographic characteristic. In short, minorities are made, not born.

of the OSU Chautauqua and this edited volume is to educate and inform, and also to create a dialogue that brings scholars, policy makers, students, and practitioners together in the goal of bridging research and practice related to resilience. We understand that a part of this work must entail beginning precisely with the complexity of history. We seek to honor the Iroquois tradition and spirit of what Chautauqua was for some by consciously extending its reach and engagement to all, and with all.

Resilience

We seek to offer a dialogue on some of the nuances of resilience. But first, why do we *need* such a concept? On the one hand, this is an asinine question. Resilience is a requirement for navigating the inevitable trials of humanity. On the other hand, some are tasked with both a greater level and a more frequent practice of resilience than others, in ways that are often patterned by inequality.

So, the question is not really why we need a concept of resilience, but why some among us need so much of it? Some populations are asked to cultivate especially high levels of resilience. Members of marginalized groups feature among those routinely tasked in such a manner. In fact, they are assumed to need instruction in fostering or building resistance in ways that can overlook and underestimate the practices of resilience they have already developed and engage routinely. Promotion and facilitation of resilience is an important good, and service providers play a critical role in its development and expansion. However, this focus can come with outsized attention on the many challenges that minoritized peoples face, to a degree that overlooks both how they forge their own paths of resistance and the varied supports they rely upon on the way.

Many of the descriptors for marginalized communities carry a negative valence. Adjectives such as deficiency, exclusion, inequality, inequity, and the like help to describe the many challenges that minoritized populations face within the United States. These challenges reiterate the importance of resilience and explain the emphasis on its facilitation and promotion among social service providers, but a lens limited in this way emphasizes a deficit model of identity. Such approaches overlook the value of internal supports, particularly the role of self and community inputs. They also motivate a tendency toward the flattening of marginalized groups. Different origin stories, histories, experiences, and struggles get subsumed under covering categories such as BIPOC, intersectionally oppressed, and minoritized, in ways that only sometimes help to illuminate different specific experiences of oppression and in/justice. As a result, marginalization itself becomes the central identifying characteristic, rather than a condition to fight against. Important elements of this fight may be shared in some instances. In other instances, difference plays a significant role. Different experiences accrue and thus different toolkits are required, leading to different cultures and practices of resilience, and even practices of and cultures of *resistance*, an approach that appears throughout the chapters that follow.

Attention across and within population diversity can highlight how the impacts of minority status might both manifest differently within sub-populations, and simultaneously serve as a source of strength. What of joy, celebration, solidarity and uplift, and the roles those conditions play in fostering resilience? Capturing the how of resilience, the particular ways in which identity functions on the spectrum from survival to thriving, is an empirical inquiry. A more nuanced view of marginalization helps us to assess inputs from both ends of the spectrum. It is precisely the interest in the how of resistance, and its accompanying forms, that brings these two conference sessions and the resulting chapters fully into conversation with one another.

Hence a dialogue on the nuances of resilience. The authors included here work in different but complementary areas. An overarching theme among them is their focus on the how of resilience, and the situating of this query in regard to the communal.

About This Volume

In Chap. 1, Singh et al. describe the empirically based components of queer and trans resilience that psychologists and other helping professions can address in their relationships with LGBTQ+ clients. In Chap. 2, Carlozzi examines the process of growth from doubt and fear to acceptance, and beyond acceptance to family resilience and advocacy among parents of transgender and gender-expansive persons in a professionally led support group. In Chap. 3, Roberts et al. explore the experience of developing LGBTQ+ resiliency within biological, legal, and fictive kinship networks among LGBTQ+ college students in the rural Midwest. In Chap. 4, Abreu et al. provide an overview of the current state of the literature about acceptance and support for Latinx LGBTQ people within their own Latinx community. In Chap. 5, Butler-Barnes presents "three Rs"—resistance, resilience, and reclaiming—as a method to promote equitable treatment for Black girls who have been systematically left out of conversations within society. In Chap. 6, Drywater-Whitekiller addresses the creation of the Indian Child Welfare Act of 1978 and its effects on American Indian/Alaska Native tribal identities. In Chap. 7, Warner explores how African American homeschooling continues a historical legacy of resilience salient to African American efforts to achieve educational freedom and excellence. In Chap. 8, Wingate introduces concepts from Black Psychology and describes a new framework for the study of Black mental health and practice. We invite the reader to join us in celebrating the ways in which multiple identities serve as sources of strength and resilience for families.

Iowa City, IA, USA — Julie M. Koch
Stillwater, OK, USA — Erica E. Townsend-Bell
West Lafayette, IN, USA — Randolph D. Hubach

Acknowledgments

We are appreciative of series editor Dr. Amanda Harrist for inviting us to chair the Chautauqua conferences in 2021 and 2022 and for her assistance in editing this volume. We would like to thank the Oklahoma State University Center for Family Resilience and Oklahoma State University College of Education and Human Sciences, Oklahoma State University College of Arts and Sciences Africana Studies, and Oklahoma State University Division of Institutional Diversity for their support of the annual Chautauqua conference. A special thanks to Dr. Brooke Tuttle and Hannah James for their vision, logistic and resource support, and camaraderie. Without them the conference would remain in the land of good, but unrealized ideas. Thanks also to all of the chapter reviewers and OSU Center for Family Resilience staff for their invaluable support. We would especially like to thank Carly Dunn, doctoral student in Human Development and Family Science at Oklahoma State University, for her assistance in understanding the importance of acknowledging Indigenous languages and traditions, and Vanessa Adams Harris, citizen of the Muscogee (Creek) Nation with African and European ancestry, and John Hope Franklin Center for Reconciliation for leading us in a session on thinking and navigating our contemporary and historic connections to the Chautauqua at the 2022 conference. We also want to acknowledge all of the contributors to this volume for giving of their time not only to present their scholarship at the conference, but also for sharing through their written chapters in this volume. Finally, we want to express our gratitude to our partners and families for their continued support of our work.

Contents

About the Series Editor

Amanda W. Harrist, (she/her), received her PhD in Child and Family Studies from the University of Tennessee, Knoxville. She is currently a Professor of Human Development and Family Science at Oklahoma State University, where she is also Associate Director for Education and Translation at the Center for Family Resilience. Her research is focused on understanding psychosocial risk and protective processes in children's social contexts, particularly the parent-child relationship and peer relations at school, where the focus is on understanding and teaching social inclusion versus social rejection and ostracism.

About the Volume Editors

Julie M. Koch, PhD, LHSP (she/they), is a Professor of Counseling Psychology in the Department of Psychological and Quantitative Foundations at the University of Iowa. Before joining the University of Iowa, she was Professor and Head of the School of Community Health Sciences, Counseling and Counseling Psychology at Oklahoma State University. Dr. Koch was a Fulbright Specialist to the Mongolia LGBT Centre in 2015, is a past American Psychological Association representative to the International Psychology Network on LGBT Issues, and has served on the American Psychological Association Committee for Global Psychology and Committee on Women in Psychology. Her interests include multicultural competence, training, and development of faculty and counseling psychologists; human rights and social justice; LGBTQ mental health and affirmative practice, especially in rural and international settings; prevention; and microaffirmation.

Erica E. Townsend-Bell, PhD (she/her/ella), is an Associate Professor of Political Science and Director of the Center for African Studies at Oklahoma State University. Dr. Townsend-Bell currently serves as a board member of the American Political Science Association's flagship journal, *The American Political Science Review*. She previously served as a member of the APSA Committee on the Status of Women, and as program section chair for the Western Political Science Association and Midwest Political Science Association annual conferences. Her areas of expertise include the politics of intersectionality, comparative race and gender politics, and social movements, especially across the Americas.

Randolph D. Hubach, PhD, MPH (he/him), is an Associate Professor of Public Health and the Director of the Sexual Health Research Lab at Purdue University. Early in his career, Dr. Hubach's research and practice experiences included serving as PI on a federally funded community-based sexual health intervention project, developing managed care programs for local public health and mental health jurisdictions, and serving in leadership positions in multiple community health coalitions and planning processes. As a behavioral scientist and public health researcher, he has gained a practical understanding of the challenges associated with the delivery of public health programs that are scientifically sound and responsive to the needs of diverse communities. Dr. Hubach's research program focuses on three key areas: (1) HIV prevention and care; (2) LGBT health disparities; and (3) rural health and the intersection of these three areas.

Contributors

Roberto L. Abreu, PhD (he/him/él), is an Assistant Professor of Counseling Psychology and the Director of the Collective Healing and Empowering VoicEs through Research and Engagement (¡Chévere!) in the Department of Psychology at the University of Florida (UF). His research explores ways in which marginalized communities resist systemic oppression and promote collective well-being. Specifically, Roberto's work has made significant contributions in two areas: (a) intersection of Latinx lesbian, gay, bisexual, transgender, and queer (LGBTQ) youth and their families and communities, and (b) transgender and gender diverse (TGD) youth and their families and communities. Roberto's work is guided by social justice values such as person-environment interactions, growth, resilience, and resistance.

Koree S. Badio, MS (she/her/hers), is a second-year Counseling Psychology PhD student at the University of Florida. She received her Bachelor of Arts in Psychology at Georgia State University and her Master of Science in Psychology at the University of Florida. Born in Atlanta, Georgia and raised in an ethnically diverse Black immigrant household, Koree is passionate about developing translational and culturally affirming healing interventions that engender psychological, spiritual, and political wellness for Black people across the Diaspora.

Olufunke Benson, MA, is a doctoral student in the Clinical Psychology program at Oklahoma State University working under the direction of Dr. LaRicka Wingate. Olufunke received her master's in Community Psychology from the University of New Haven, Connecticut, and her Bachelor's in Psychology from the University of Ibadan, Nigeria. Olufunke's research interests focuses on examining culturally specific risk and protective factors that can be found within Black and African American communities that can be used to mitigate suicidality and other mental health disorders among the population.

Sheretta T. Butler-Barnes, PhD, is an Associate Professor of Social Work at Washington University in St. Louis (WUSTL). A developmental psychologist and quantitative methodologist, Butler-Barnes' line of research includes examining how Black youth draw on individual and cultural assets and resources to thrive despite challenges to their identities from structural, individual, and cultural racism. Her expertise and scholarly work is on Black children and youth, risk and resilience, academic achievement, and wellbeing. Butler-Barnes also has extensive experience in youth programming as it pertains to Black adolescent girls.

Alfred F. Carlozzi, EdD, is a licensed health service psychologist, licensed marital and family therapist, and Professor Emeritus at Oklahoma State University (OSU). He retired from OSU in 2019, after serving 40 years on the OSU faculty. Administrative positions he held at OSU include interim department head, school head, associate dean/interim dean of the Graduate College, and for his last 13 years with OSU, he served as Professor and Director of the OSU-Tulsa Counseling Center. Awards he received include the OSU Regents Distinguished Teaching Award, OSU-Tulsa Outstanding Teaching Award, Distinguished Researcher Award, and Leadership and Service Excellence Award. For more than 10 years, Dr. Carlozzi has served on committees and/or the board of directors for Mental Health Association Oklahoma and as co-leader of the support group for parents of transgender persons at the Dennis R. Neill Equality Center. He has conducted numerous presentations on gender affirming counseling for transgender and gender expansive persons. He is co-editor of the book *Transgender and Gender Diverse Persons: A Handbook for Service Providers, Educators, and Families*.

Déjà N. Clement, MS, MPH, is a Clinical Psychology Doctoral Candidate at Oklahoma State University and incoming intern at Massachusetts General Hospital/Harvard Medical School. Her research and clinical work take an interdisciplinary approach combining both public health and clinical psychology. She aims to understand and mitigate the impact of systemic oppression and discrimination on health behaviors and health outcomes for minoritized communities through the development of culturally responsive and community-based interventions.

Virginia Drywater-Whitekiller (United Keetoowah Band of Cherokee Indians), EdD, MSW, is a Professor of Social Work at Northeastern State University in Tahlequah, Oklahoma. In addition to full-time teaching, Dr. Drywater-Whitekiller pursues an active research agenda utilizing the theory of cultural resilience as applied to American Indian/Alaska Native/First Nations population issues such as microaggressions, higher education retention, identity, and Indian child welfare. In 2009 she was selected as a Smithsonian Community Scholar conducting research at the Smithsonian Archives in Suitland, Maryland. More recently, she served as the 2018–2019 Fulbright Canada Jarislowsky Research Chair in Aboriginal Studies at Vancouver Island University, British Columbia.

Rebekah Estevez, PhD (she/her), is an Assistant Professor at Georgia Southern University in the PsyD, Clinical Psychology program. Bekah's teaching interests include multicultural psychology, psychotherapy skills, advocacy, and helping students learn the art and science of psychotherapy grounded in strengths-based, culturally responsive approaches. Believing in the potential for psychology to attenuate human suffering based in racism, heteronormativity, and other axes of oppression, she works to use her privilege as a white queer cisgender woman to explore the lived experiences of risk and resilience of those living at the intersections of oppressive systems. Broadly, Bekah's research interests include resilience, the impact of intersecting systems of oppression on mental health, best psychotherapy practices for working with the LGBTQ+ community, and bridging scholarly work and practice towards improving the field of psychology's role in mitigating disparate health outcomes experienced in Black and Latinx LGBTQ+ communities.

Regina Finan, PhD, NCC (she/her), is an Assistant Professor in the Clinical Mental Health Counseling program at Agnes Scott College. Her career working with college students, experience with mental health counseling, and training as a counselor educator provide her with a unique perspective on the education and training of students in mental health disciplines. Her research includes an examination of race-based discrimination, multicultural and social justice training and pedagogy, and multiracial identity. Dr. Finan is committed to providing and promoting education, engagement, research, community-building, and resources pertaining to the needs and experiences of diverse students and communities.

Sarah Haueisen, MA (they/them), is a rising fifth-year doctoral student in the Counseling Psychology Ph.D. program at Western Michigan University. Sarah's dissertation focuses on increasing the multicultural competence of White school counselors and school counselors-in-training. They hope to use their work to raise awareness of barriers to multicultural counseling and increase white counselors' comfort in providing care to racial or ethnically marginalized populations. Sarah will begin their pre-doctoral internship at the University of Colorado-Boulder in Fall 2023.

Aaron D. Jones, MA (he/him), is a recent alumnus of the Counseling Psychology MA program at Western Michigan University. He has wide-ranging interests in mental health, community, and service work with Black and other communities of color and queer people of color (QPOC) issues, focusing on general well-being and health. After graduate school, Aaron returned to his native Baltimore to begin a career focused on promoting the welfare and protection of clients while promoting ethical standards within the profession.

Julio A. Martin, MFT (he/him), is a rising third-year doctoral student at the University of Florida, Counseling Psychology program. Prior to joining the Counseling Psychology program, Julio received a bachelor's degree with honors, research distinction, in psychology from Florida International University and a master's degree in Marriage and Family Therapy from the University of Miami. Julio identifies as a cis-gender, queer, first-generation Latino Cuban-American man. Currently, Julio examines the role of cultural values in the parenting practices of Latinx LGBTQ+ families and is overall interested in studying the parenting practices of Latinx families.

Vanessa Oliphant, MS, is a Doctoral Candidate in the Clinical Psychology program at Oklahoma State University working under the direction of Dr. LaRicka Wingate. Vanessa received her master's in Community Psychology from Florida A&M University and her bachelor's in African American Studies from the University of California, Berkeley. Vanessa's research interests focus on examining risk and protective factors for Black women's experiences with suicidal ideation.

Tangela Roberts, PhD, is an Assistant Professor of Counselor Education and Counseling Psychology at Western Michigan University. She received her PhD in Counseling Psychology from the University of Massachusetts, Boston. She earned her undergraduate degree in Psychology and Women's Studies at St. John's University and a master's degree in Community Counseling from the University of Wisconsin-Madison. Dr. Roberts has clinical experience with adolescents and young adults at both college counseling centers and community mental health clinics. Her primary line of research focuses on predictors of mental health outcomes for Black LGBTQ+ individuals. Specifically, she focuses on the impact of community supports and microaggressions. Additionally, she analyzes how queer people of color participate in their communities, activism, and receive other forms of social support.

Anneliese A. Singh, PhD, LPC (she/they), serves as Chief Diversity Officer at Tulane University and is a Professor in the School of Social Work with a joint appointment in the Department of Psychology. Dr. Singh's scholarship and community organizing explores racial healing and racial justice, as well as the resilience, trauma, and identity development experiences of queer and trans people, with a focus on young people and BIPOC people. Dr. Singh is the author of *The Racial Healing Handbook* and *The Queer and Trans Resilience Workbook*. Dr. Singh founded the Trans Resilience Project to translate her LGBTQ+ research findings into school and community-based change efforts, including NIH-funded work with trans and nonbinary people in Project AFFIRM.

Tatyana Smith, MA (she/her), is a rising fifth-year doctoral student in the Counseling Psychology PhD program at Western Michigan University. Tatyana's dissertation focuses on Black men's positionality within interpersonal systems and exposure to multiple systems of oppression (i.e., social, cultural, political, contextual, and historical) in relation to experiences with childhood sexual abuse, romantic relationships, and masculinity. She hopes to use her research to create social wellness programs that promote the relationship functioning of Black couples whose male partners have histories of childhood sexual abuse. After completing her PhD,

Tatyana wants to work as a faculty member at a Historically Black College and University (HBCU).

Stacie L. Warner, MEd, is a doctoral student in the Social Foundations of Education (SCFD) program at Oklahoma State University (OSU). Her research and scholarship address Intersectional Disabilities and African American homeschooling. Stacie is a graduate of the University of Central Oklahoma (UCO) with a Master of Education degree. She has over 10 years of experience in adult education and training. She is also a veteran of the US Air Force.

LaRicka R. Wingate, PhD, is a Professor of Psychology and Africana Studies affiliate faculty at Oklahoma State University. Dr. Wingate is dedicated to Black-centered mental health research. She is particularly interested in those strengths thought to serve as protective factors for African Americans and other marginalized groups. She examines risk and protective factors that may be particularly salient to Black suicide and mental health, including the impact of acculturation, racial microaggressions, historical trauma, racial/ethnic discrimination, and intersectionality. Dr. Wingate has published more than 75 scholarly publications that have appeared in high quality academic journals.

Grace Yensch, MA (they/them), is a rising fourth-year doctoral student in the Counseling Psychology PhD program at Western Michigan University. Grace's dissertation explores methods to improve counselor competency when working with transgender and gender non-conforming (TGNC) clients. They are also interested in the intersection of race and LGBTQ+ identity among individuals with a privileged racial identity and a marginalized sexual orientation or gender identity (i.e., White LGBTQ+ individuals). Grace hopes to use their research to further best practices when working with TGNC clients and to further clinical research exploring racism within White LGBTQ+ communities. They mentioned personal experiences of viewing LGBTQ+ communities as majority White and full of White supremacy culture.

Chapter 1
Queer and Trans Resilience: Moving from Affirmation to Liberation in Our Collective Healing

Anneliese A. Singh, Regina Finan, and Rebekah Estevez

In queer and 2STNB (two-spirit, trans, nonbinary) health, development, counseling, and psychology, the helping professions have often mirrored the very societal values that drive heterosexism and other intersectional oppressions. For instance, the roots of colonization and anti-Black racism in the land we now call the United States of America erased variances of gender and sexuality present in Indigenous communities and left us with incorrect binary notions of gender and similarly oppressive structures of heteronormative sexuality (Singh, 2016, 2020). Therefore, we are looking to our helping professions for healing for our queer and 2STNB communities, families, and individuals when these professions have not embarked on intentional decolonization efforts (Mosley et al., 2020; Singh et al., 2020a, b). What we are left with is an "upside down" state, where queer and 2STNB helping professionals and our allies and accomplices lead the work of naming embedded intersectional oppressions within our disciplines, leaving us in a state of simultaneously fighting both within and outside of the metaphorical walls of our professions to fight for freedom, justice, and our liberation. This is clear when you look back at the trajectory of queer and 2STNB health, counseling, and psychology. There was first the emergence of "affirmative" practices with our communities. We affirmed that our communities existed, were real, deserved services, and needed affirmation of our humanity. For decades we continued this affirmative work (ACA, 2010; Singh &

A. A. Singh (✉)
Tulane University, New Orleans, LA, USA
e-mail: anneliese@tulane.edu

R. Finan
University of West Georgia, Carrollton, GA, USA

R. Estevez
Georgia Southern University, Statesboro, GA, USA

J. M. Koch et al. (eds.), *Identity as Resilience in Minoritized Communities*, Emerging Issues in Family and Individual Resilience,
https://doi.org/10.1007/978-3-031-38977-1_1

Dickey, 2017), which was critical to engaging multicultural and social justice counseling competencies with our communities.

At the same time, a longer conversation about abolition and liberation was taking place in the world outside of the helping professions where colonization and anti-Black racism had taken place (Singh, 2020). These conversations started to drive counseling and psychology to question our white, western roots and to acknowledge the roots of mental health healing in multiple other parts of the world – including the continent of Africa and BIPOC (Black, Indigenous, People of Color) countries around the world. Through these conversations, we began to question the aims of affirmative practice – not that we wanted to throw away the importance of affirming our queer and 2STNB identities and lived realities in an oppressive sociopolitical state – but to name the larger aims of liberation (Singh et al., 2020a, b). As Singh (2020, pp. 1112–1113) notes,

> We all have a personal experience of liberation. It is the feeling deep in our bones when we are free from all the internalized messages we were taught of who we were supposed to be and the expansion we feel when we transform these messages into critical consciousness to act upon the world and change it.

The project of working toward liberation for all people who experience oppression is one that frees all of us along the way. Liberation is a psychological construct, but it only has meaning when we enact it. Liberation moves us beyond the debates of whether or not we should engage in advocacy and social justice, and moves us to envision the world we want to leave behind as counseling psychologists and actively build towards that world.

Think about it. What would a world free of racism, sexism, heterosexism, classism, ableism, anti-immigrant sentiment, and other oppressions *"look like?"* Building a counseling psychology of liberation helps us dream that this new world can not only exist, but that there are also specific action steps as counseling psychologists that we can take right now to work towards that goal; and, this means "liberation" should take its place alongside our other hallmark counseling psychology values of lifespan and career development, prevention and wellness, multiculturalism, and social justice.

Keeping in mind this definition of liberation of both a moment – and a series of moments – of actions and processes of undoing heterosexist and other intersectional oppressive learnings, in this article we examine the lived realities of queer and 2STNB communities in our helping professions and how to best serve them moving from affirmative to liberatory practices. In this chapter, we alternate between using terms such as "queer and trans" to "LGBTQ+" and "queer and 2STNB" to describe our incredible community and we look forward to all of the new ways our community will describe ourselves that have not yet been articulated in word or print.

1.1 Queer and Trans Risk and Resilience: What We Are Fighting and How We Fight Back

As previously described, using an intersectional (Crenshaw, 1989) and minority stress theory (Brooks, 1981; Meyer, 2015) framework, we know that LGBTQ+ individuals experience unique identity-based stress that negatively impacts health and well-being due to the intersection of cisnormativity, heteronormativity, and subsequent prejudice, stigma, and discrimination. While our focus in this chapter intentionally uses a strengths-based perspective, it is important to review the extant literature regarding salient identity-based minority stressors to health and well-being against which queer and 2STNB communities build resilience. To name the very real impacts of racism, heteronormativity, cisnormativity, ableism, adultism, and the myriad of other systems of oppression bearing down on queer and 2STNB communities is to name the insidious ways white body supremacy culture seeks to de-story LGBTQ+ individuals and communities, both from within and outside the LGBTQ+ community itself (Menakem, 2017; Parmenter et al., 2021; Singh et al., 2020a, b).

Importantly, we recognize and honor the heterogeneity of the "LGBTQ+ community," which is often a microcosm of the majority culture due to power imbalances that center white, cisgender, gay men (Koech et al., 2022; McConnell et al., 2018; Noyola et al., 2020). Therefore, it is important to take into account the particular contexts, power structures, and experiences of microcommunities within the broader LGBTQ+ community when discussing both risk and resilience. For the purposes of this chapter, we will focus on two particularly vulnerable yet resilient subcommunities – LGBTQ+ BIPOC and LGBTQ+ youth and young adults. Importantly, while cisgender LGB and 2STNB communities' experiences of risk and resilience can sometimes overlap, the nature of cissexism and heteronormativity operate differently for cisgender LGB and 2STNB individuals. Due to page constraints for this chapter, we will include relevant research and discussion regarding the entirety of the LGBTQ+ community including information specific and unique to cisgender and 2STNB individuals.

1.2 LGBTQ+ BIPOC Communities

LGBTQ+ BIPOC individuals often must navigate risks to well-being from within their racial/ethnic community, the broader majority culture, and within the LGBTQ+ community itself (Follins et al., 2014; Schmitz et al., 2020a, b; Stone et al., 2020; Sutter & Perrin, 2016). While it is erroneous and reductionary to assume that BIPOC cultural communities are more heterosexist and/or cissexist than white cultural communities (Abreu & Gonzalez, 2020; Robinson, 2018; Velez et al., 2015), the impact of European colonization integrated with many BIPOC cultural values is such that LGBTQ+ BIPOC individuals can experience difficulty navigating family of origin and community relationships that usually are a source of support and resilience against racism (e.g., *machismo*, *marianismo* gender roles in the Latinx community; see Abreu et al., 2021a, b, c, this volume; Estevez, 2022; Noyola et al., 2020). Salient risks to well-being experienced by LGBTQ+ BIPOC due to the intersection of racism, cisnormativity, and heteronormativity include within-ethnic/racial cultural discrimination (e.g., Ball et al., 2021; Ghabrial, 2017); familial rejection and non-affirmation of identities (e.g., Salerno et al., 2022; Sutter & Perrin, 2016; Yadegarfard et al., 2014); employment discrimination, housing insecurity, and other socioeconomic instabilities (e.g., James et al., 2016; Mahowald, 2021); high rates of trauma and interpersonal violence (e.g., Fitzgerald, 2017); barriers to healthcare access (e.g., Casanova-Perez et al., 2021); and the stress of navigating concealment of identity and outness strategies within and outside their racial/ethnic community (e.g., Lockett et al., 2022; Sutter & Perrin, 2016). These risks to well-being show up in LGBTQ BIPOC people's lives through negative mental health, drug abuse, high blood pressure, and other negative health impacts (e.g., Drazdowski et al., 2016; Garcia & Kijak, 2021; Garcia & Serpas, 2021; James et al., 2016).

However, the story does not end here. A growing body of research has identified resilience processes cultivated and enacted by LGBTQ+ BIPOC community members which attenuate the negative impact of the above-mentioned risks to well-being. Perhaps one of the most salient of these resilience processes is the cultivation of community, through which LGBTQ+ BIPOC individuals gain access to tangible (e.g., knowledge of affirming healthcare providers, connection with housing options) and intangible (e.g., positive regard, affirmation of identity, acceptance) resilience resources (Abreu et al., 2021a, b, c; Hudson & Romanelli, 2020; Meyer, 2015; Singh, 2017; Singh & McKleroy, 2011). Importantly, through communion with similar others, LGBTQ+ BIPOC individuals engage in consciousness-raising regarding the intersecting systems of oppression negatively impacting themselves and their community, which often leads to engagement with activism and advocacy efforts (Parmenter et al., 2021; Singh et al., 2011). Also important to note is the essential importance of LGBTQ+ BIPOC individuals to connect with "microcommunities" that are reflective of the LGBTQ+ BIPOC individuals' own intersecting identities and subsequent needs that cannot be as well met by the larger often white and cisnormative LGBTQ+ community (e.g., immigrant, trans, Latinx; Abreu et al., 2021a, b, c). Oftentimes, giving back and helping similar others navigate experiences of oppression and gain access to resources is itself an aspect of resilience for LGBTQ+ BIPOC individuals (Cerezo et al., 2014; Estevez, 2022; Hudson & Romanelli, 2020). Through connecting with community in these various ways, LGBTQ+ BIPOC individuals cultivate aspects of internal resilience such as hope for the future, deconstructing religion and reconstructing personally meaningful faith and spirituality, developing pride in one's racialized LGBTQ+ identity, and making healthy decisions to navigate family and peer relationships (Estevez, 2022; Noyola et al., 2020; Singh & McKleroy, 2011).

1.3 LGBTQ+ Youth and Young Adults

LGBTQ+ youth and young adults (in the research reviewed here, between the ages of 13 and 28) are another vulnerable yet resilient microcommunity within the broader LGBTQ+ community. A robust body of literature shows that LGBTQ+ youth and young adults experience alarmingly high rates of suicidal ideation and/or attempts (e.g., Johns et al., 2020), disproportionate rates of mental health disorders and psychological distress (e.g., Almeida et al., 2009), substance use and abuse (e.g., Coulter et al., 2016; Mereish, 2019), engagement in non-suicidal self-injury behaviors (e.g., Taliaferro & Muehlenkamp, 2017), and are at high risk of dropping out of school and being pushed into the school-to-prison pipeline (e.g., Snapp et al., 2015). Perhaps one of the largest negative outcomes of risk to well-being is the public health crisis of disproportionate rates of LGBTQ+ youth and young adults experiencing housing insecurity (Baams et al., 2019; Morton et al., 2018). These risk outcomes are due to rampant experiences of discrimination, prejudice, rejection, and victimization from a variety of contexts within LGBTQ+ youths' lives, such as school administrators, online contexts, peers, police, churches, family of origin, and teachers (Coulter et al., 2016; Johns et al., 2020; Lardier et al., 2020; McBride, 2021; Robinson, 2020; Roe, 2017; Snapp et al., 2015). Due to the impact of cisnormativity and racism, LGBTQ+ BIPOC youth and young adults and 2STNB youth and young adults experience higher rates of the aforementioned risk experiences and negative outcomes than their cisgender and/or white counterparts (Green et al., 2022; Mallory & Russell, 2021; McBride, 2021). Importantly, in their exploration of the resilience of 2STNB youth of color, Singh (2013) named and explored the impact of adultism on the unique experiences of oppression and risk in 2STNB youth of color's lives. They argue that adultism, or the power adult caregivers wield over 2STNB youth's lives regarding gender identity, expression, and sexuality, is a salient risk to well-being that 2STNB youth, and likely all LGBTQ+ youth, must contend with (Singh, 2013).

Despite pervasive attempts to staunch LGBTQ+ youth and young adults' well-being at the social, familial, and eventually intrapersonal levels, LGBTQ+ youth and young adults resist, persist, and thrive. Within school environments, the presence and accessibility of supportive administrators, teachers, policies, and support groups collectively and individually create supportive and affirming school environments, which are essential to LGBTQ+ youth well-being (Asakura, 2019; Hillier et al., 2020). These supportive individuals and contexts are especially important for the resilience of LGBTQ+ youth and young adults who experience familial rejection or unsupportive households. When parents or parental figures (biological or foster care/shelter caregivers) offer support, affirmation, and unconditional love, LGBTQ+ youth experience positive well-being, empowerment, and internalized positive beliefs regarding their identity (González-Álvarez et al., 2022; Travers et al., 2022). Additionally, while peers can often be a source of bullying and victimization, fostering relationships with supportive peers – especially fellow LGBTQ+ peers – is also a salient source of resilience and strength for LGBTQ+ youth and young adults

(Asakura, 2017, 2019; Schmitz & Tyler, 2019). For LGBTQ+ BIPOC youth, connecting with other LGBTQ+ BIPOC community is also especially important in order for individuals to be able to feel accepted, affirmed, and understood in all of their identity complexities (Singh, 2013). An important way that LGBTQ+ youth and young adults can access supportive individuals and environments is through social media, which offers LGBTQ+ youth and young adults the opportunity to connect with mentors, role models, and therefore begin to envision future life experiences and opportunities that may not exist within their immediate contexts (Asakura, 2017; Craig et al., 2015; Singh, 2013). Also, because of the disproportionate number of LGBTQ+ youth experiencing housing insecurity, research has highlighted that accessing tangible resources such as housing or financial security, medical providers with appropriate knowledge and skills, and at times the ability to change locations and/or school environments are other important sources of resilience (Goldenberg et al., 2021; Travers et al., 2022).

1.4 Queer and 2STNB Affirming Practices

Several competencies have been created to engender an understanding of relevant considerations specific to LGBTQ+ individuals and communities (American Counseling Association [ACA], 2010; American Psychological Association [APA], 2012; APA, 2015; Harper et al., 2013; National Association of Social Workers [NASW], 2015a, b). Additional competencies, ethical codes, and standards affirm a commitment to diversity, social justice, and advocacy for marginalized groups (ACA, 2014; APA, 2010; Council for the Accreditation of Counseling and Related Programs [CACREP], 2016; Counselors for Social Justice [CSJ], 2011; National Organization of Human Services, 2015; Ratts et al., 2016). These resources provide us with a framework to better understand and support individuals located at the margins of our society, focusing our attention to language, definitions, and guidelines for personal and professional competence. Collectively, these works join with scholarly literature to address a glaring need for moving beyond interventions and practices to support well-being for queer and 2STNB folx; rather, it is incumbent upon society to create and preserve liberatory circumstances for individuals identifying as part of this community.

Research consistently informs us that queer and 2STNB folx are at risk for numerous emotional, mental, and physical health challenges (Toomey et al., 2017; White Hughto et al., 2015). However, it is necessary to also recognize that there is incredible strength and resilience in this community. Individuals who identify as members of LGBTQ+ communities demonstrate considerable resilience in the face of stigma (White Hughto et al., 2015), political oppression and marginalization (Brown & Keller, 2018), and most recently, a global pandemic (Gonzalez et al., 2021). A growing body of literature indicates methods of affirming practices that are beneficial to queer and 2STNB folx (Bettergarcia et al., 2021; Goldenberg et al., 2019; Knutson et al., 2022; Leland & Stockwell, 2019; Matsuno, 2019). We bear a responsibility to explicate affirming practices and conditions that contribute to their well-being. Affirming practices are those which create the possibility for queer and 2STNB folx to experience the same value as a human being, with the capacity for self-agency and access to resources, that cisgender people enjoy (Leland & Stockwell, 2019). Operating from a strengths-based approach grounded in resilience and well-being is essential to promote these practices and conditions (ACA, 2010). When individuals with these identities are not afforded affirmation, they instead experience a lack of respect and self-autonomy; this can damage their sense of self, resulting in trauma (Barr et al., 2021). However, inclusive policies and practices can engender a greater sense of belongingness (Goldberg et al., 2019) and should occur at multiple systemic levels [e.g., micro/individual, mezzo/interpersonal, and macro/structural] (Leland & Stockwell, 2019; Matsuno, 2019; White Hughto et al., 2015).

Practitioners and helping professionals must engage in honest and rigorous self-reflection and self-assessment on their attitudes and behaviors, knowledge, skills, and actions related to LGBTQ+ issues and concerns (ACA, 2010; Harper et al., 2013; Ratts et al., 2016; Singh & McKleroy, 2011). An integral component of this work for professionals is interrogating their own gender identity journey in an effort to connect more deeply and personally with this essential element for queer and 2STNB folx (Singh et al., 2014). Adopting a practice of cultural humility can support practitioners in these efforts (Leland & Stockwell, 2019). There is insufficient data to adequately measure professional competence in working with queer and 2STNB people, but existing data suggest considerable room for improvement (Bettergarcia et al., 2021; McCullough et al., 2017). For mental health counselors, counseling psychologists, and other health professionals, training designed to enhance competence in working with this population should also be paired with clinical supervision to reduce bias and increase affirming behaviors and skills (Lelutiu-Weinberger et al., 2022). Additionally, professionals who work with this population must remain knowledgeable about legislation and policies that either restrict or protect the rights of queer and 2STNB individuals (Abreu et al., 2021a, b, c). Education, training, and practice will benefit from an intersectional framework, addressing interlocking systems of oppression that are pervasive in the lives of queer and 2STNB folx of color (Parmenter et al., 2021).

1.5 Affirming Queer and 2STNB Theoretical Frameworks

Operating solely within traditional theoretical frameworks, promulgated by primarily white cisgender European men, may not best serve queer and 2STNB people (Singh et al., 2020a, b).

Theories are essential to helping professions, as they help practitioners to develop a framework for conceptualizing clients, patients, students, and families in a way that is consistent with a practitioner's own values (Drapela, 1990). Intersectionality and relational cultural theory (RCT) (Baker, 1986) are two affirming frameworks that can promote healthy, inclusive, and productive work with queer and 2STNB clients.

Intersectionality was conceptualized by Kimberlé Crenshaw, a Black feminist and critical legal scholar, as a way to examine the compounding effects of multiple oppressions at the intersection of race and gender (Crenshaw, 1989). Similarly, queer and 2STNB folx must maneuver uniquely nuanced and complex intersections and interactions of oppression and resilience (Chan, 2018). This is especially true for 2STND and queer folx of color. Intersectionality is especially useful as an affirming lens for culturally responsive therapeutic work by critiquing how systems of power and privilege operate within the lives of marginalized people (Abreu et al., 2021a, b, c; Adames et al., 2018). Further, an intersectional framework can assist in interrogating how systems of oppression are perpetuated within the LGBTQ+ community (Parmenter et al., 2021).

Pioneered by the work of Jean Miller Baker (1986), relational cultural theory (RCT) has increasingly been identified as an affirming theoretical framework in supporting queer and 2STNB individuals (Chan et al., 2021; Flores & Sheely-Moore, 2020; Patton & Reicherzer, 2010; Singh et al., 2020a, b; Singh & Moss, 2016). This framework is a relational approach, attending to how complex power dynamics create and maintain connections or disconnections for individuals (Comstock et al., 2008; Jordan, 2001). The marginalization and oppression queer and 2STNB folx are subjected to threaten their emotional, psychological, relational, and physical well-being (Jordan, 2008). Affirming practices through an RCT approach can include examining and processing themes of cultural complexity, isolation, shame, relational competence, mutual empathy, and power in relationships (Singh & Moss, 2016); exploring authenticity, vulnerability, and radical respect during a process of counseling for gender transition counseling (Patton & Reicherzer, 2010); deconstructing the experience of intersecting forms of oppression for LGBTQ+ older adults of color (Chan et al., 2021); and implementing RCT tenets to explore societally imposed stigma and the ensuing impact on relational wellness for LGBTQ college students (Flores & Sheely-Moore, 2020).

1.6 Sociopolitical Considerations and Affirming Social Support

Recent policies and bills restrict 2STNB youth from sports, limit their access to healthcare, and exclude them from gender-affirming bathrooms and forms of identification (American Civil Liberties Union [ACLU], 2022). These are insidious forms of oppression which negatively impact queer and 2STNB folx, especially people of color, resulting in depression, anxiety, suicidal ideation, and other harmful consequences (Abreu et al., 2022). Specifically, during the presidency of Donald Trump, immigrant Latinx 2STNB individuals experienced multiple oppressions which created an environment of hostility associated with rhetoric and policies

(Abreu et al., 2021a, b, c), which can signal permission to groups and individuals willing to enact emotional, psychological, political, and physical harm to queer and 2STNB folx (Flaskerud & Lesser, 2018). Some 2STNB individuals may have both negative and positive perceptions of current sociopolitical experiences. For example, there are positive experiences related to increased representations of trans people in media, expansion in gender-affirming care providers, language, and access to documentation (Bockting et al., 2020). However, resistance has accompanied some of these expansions, resulting in increased discrimination, violence, and bills and policies restricting advances made to support the mental health and well-being of 2STNB individuals (Bockting et al., 2020).

Society increasingly exhibits anti-2STNB bias and sends messages of non-affirmation to individuals who identify as queer and 2STNB, which may promote Post-Traumatic Stress Disorder symptoms (Barr et al., 2021). Therefore, affirming social support for individuals in this community is essential. Adaptive relationships are instrumental in supporting resilience for 2STNB communities (Bockting et al., 2020; Budge et al., 2014; Gorman et al., 2020). These relationships are necessary in all areas of life including with family, friends, educators, healthcare providers, and various service providers. Multiple spaces can be dangerous for queer and 2STNB folx – many that they cannot avoid, such as school. Ideally, students in education training programs would be introduced to content, concepts, and strategies to create trans-inclusive spaces in schools (DePedro et al., 2016), but this is often where these students are victimized (Russell et al., 2011). Social support may be particularly important for young people, and especially LGBTQ+ youth of color, as they may be trying to successfully connect with a community (Singh, 2013) during a time of significant developmental growth (Eccles & Roeser, 2011).

Members of social support networks for queer and 2STNB folx can contact legislators and policymakers about legislation and policies that are harmful (Abreu et al., 2022). Some specific recommendations include (a) asking those with state and federal power to not politicize healthcare for queer and 2STNB folx, (b) decriminalizing healthcare for these individuals, (c) enacting policies and laws which prevent and address violence and prejudice against this population, and (d) investing in more education about queer and 2STNB people and related concerns (Abreu et al., 2022). Gay-Straight Alliances may provide students with additional social support and have been associated with a reduction in bullying in schools (Day et al., 2020). Schools with policies that support LGBTQ+ students can provide students with a sense of safety and adult allyship (Day et al., 2020). Additionally, it is important for youth to have social support systems that include family of origin, family of choice, friends, and the broader community (e.g., healthcare providers, educators) (Katz-Wise et al., 2020).

With regard to older queer and 2STNB adults, some initial data suggest that legislation restricting queer and 2STNB rights may result in negative mental health outcomes (Horne et al., 2022), as well as the long-term impact of this stress on mental and physical health. We also have limited knowledge on differential mental health outcomes for queer and 2STNB folx in different developmental stages. In fact, there is a paucity of scholarly work investigating experiences for older

LGBTQ+ adults (Chaney & Whitman, 2020). Finally, it is necessary to engage in intersectional frameworks to better understand experiences of multiple marginalized queer and 2STNB people and contextual considerations of multifaceted experiences (Layland et al., 2020). For example, while queer and 2STNB BIPOC may feel their families reject their gender identity, they may also experience acceptance and support for their racial/ethnic identity (Singh & McKleroy, 2011).

1.7 Implications for Understanding Family Resilience

It may be especially important for LGBTQ+ youth to have familial support during a time when they are navigating stressful developmental life stages in addition to the complexities of development related to other salient identities (e.g., sexual orientation, gender identity, race/ethnicity, ability status) (Chan, 2018; Needham & Austin, 2010). However, families may reject queer and 2STNB family members due to their gender identity, gender expression, or stigma associated with HIV/AIDS (Hailey et al., 2020). This may be especially true in BIPOC families (Hailey et al., 2020) and religious families (Vanderwaal et al., 2017). When these youth lack familial support, there may be negative outcomes related to their well-being (Needham & Austin, 2010).

Conversely, many families support their queer and 2STNB family members and are experiencing fear, anxiety, and anger in response to recent efforts to restrict gender-affirming healthcare (Abreu et al., 2021a, b, c). Parental figures for these youth understand the harmful effects of these actions (Abreu et al., 2022) and may use various strategies in response, such as (a) engaging in forms of activism and advocacy, (b) creating opportunities for education, (c) seeking support, and (d) making plans to relocate (Abreu et al., 2021a, b, c). In many cases, parents may not initially support their children (Katz-Wise et al., 2020; Roe, 2017). In fact, families and other social support system members may feel overwhelmed and hopeless about how to cope with the issues impacting queer and 2STNB individuals they care for. Research indicates that families may need gender-affirming resources and strategies for how to support queer and 2STNB youth (Andrzewjewski et al., 2020). Specific examples include (a) emotional support when youth come out, (b) creating space for youth to talk about gender, social, legal, and medical support, and (c) using gender-affirming pronouns and their chosen name (Andrzewjewski et al., 2020). Many families do not have the ability to change their geographic location; however, it is important to recognize that some settings are not as conducive to affirming youth well-being as others (Katz-Wise et al., 2020), resulting in isolation and limited opportunities to form meaningful and supportive relationships.

In an effort to connect with others, individuals with these identities may create a chosen family with other queer and 2STNB folx and allies (Hailey et al., 2020). These chosen families can be a protective factor, performing various caretaking functions for one another such as medical support, emotional support, and mutual aid (Levin et al., 2020). In many cases, chosen family may not actually replace one's biological family, but rather complement it (Hull & Ortyl, 2019). Ultimately, it can be helpful for practitioners to establish a good working relationship with parents and relevant caregivers. Family counseling may provide an opportunity to process feelings and identify strategies to address internalized heterosexism and other intersectional oppressions. Utilizing an intersectional family framework (Schmitz et al., 2020a, b), whereby multiple identities (e.g., race/ethnicity, gender identity, sexual orientation, religion, ability) are considered within the context of oppression, privilege, and resilience, may be useful.

Focusing on individual and family resilience is an important affirming practice (Singh & McKleroy, 2011). Queer and 2STNB folx are entrenched in deficit narratives which can overwhelm them and reduce them to simply living a problematic existence. While exploring negative experiences is necessary, it is also essential to examine growth, resilience, and resistance in their journey (Singh et al., 2011; Singh & McKleroy, 2011). Resilience in the form of pride in racial/ethnic and gender identities, as well as developing self-efficacy in traversing related oppressive experiences, is particularly salient (Singh & McKleroy, 2011). As a reminder, resilience is an important aspect of queer and 2STNB resistance to societal oppression. Individual and/or family resilience is developed in response to adversity, which an anti-queer and anti-2STNB society intentionally creates conditions supporting cis-heteronormativity. We also believe that when we understand resilience-as-resistance is a core part of queer and 2STNB healing, we are moving toward more liberatory processes of healing where client freedom is the ultimate aim and goal.

1.8 Moving Towards Liberatory Practices

Thus, while multicultural and social justice competency practices have served us well, it is time to adopt more liberatory approaches. This approach requires those in helping professions to refrain from asking queer and 2STNB folx to adapt and develop resilience; it requires all of us to examine cisgender privilege and heteronormativity within a more expansive and intersectional framework inclusive of white supremacy, racism, classism, and adultism (Parmenter et al., 2021; Singh, 2016; Singh, 2020). Queer and 2STNB folx continue to be stigmatized, othered, and subjected to unnecessary and dehumanizing barriers (Flaskerud & Lesser, 2018). Engaging in advocacy to advance rights and safety for these individuals can advance a liberation approach (ACA, 2018; Singh et al., 2020a, b); this approach encompasses multiculturally oriented attitudes and beliefs, knowledge, skills, and actions (Ratts et al., 2016).

Training programs continue to lack adequate education to prepare helping professionals and educators in gender-affirming practices for queer and 2STNB people (Singh, 2016). This is considerably problematic, as a significant stressor for individuals in this community can be the burden of constantly educating others (Gorman et al., 2020). To further reject adherence to binary conceptualizations of gender, we can promote acceptance of an individual's right to choose their own gender expression without having to conform to "passing" as a specific gender as a strategy for safety (Anderson et al., 2020). This is not a universal experience, however. Many individuals in this community want their gender expression to match their gender identity and adopting a radically inclusive 2STNB agency framework urges society to release heteronormative and cisnormative expectations. Radical inclusivity demands that we move beyond performative inclusion and truly create spaces of safety and belonging (Bain et al., 2016). Ultimately, we must listen to queer and 2STNB people and intentionally center their voices (Goldberg et al., 2019).

Liberation is a process and outcome of resisting oppression to achieve psychopolitical (a confluence of psychological and political) wellness (Mosley et al., 2021; Prilleltensky, 2003, 2008; Singh, 2020). Activism, optimism, and resistance are critical elements of liberatory practices. While activism experiences may be stressful, they can also engender empowerment and enhance a sense of community and self-worth (Bockting et al., 2020; Singh et al., 2011; Singh & McKleroy, 2011). Notably, activism may support well-being, particularly for youth most impacted by multiple oppressions (Frost et al., 2019). Optimism can be an essential element of resistance and hope (Singh et al., 2011; Singh & McKleroy, 2011). Centering, exploring, and practicing resistance can help all of us to revolutionize current oppressive conditions (Mosley et al., 2020, 2021). Queer and 2STNB individuals and families may also benefit from a greater sense of agency and critical consciousness related to gender identity, gender expression, and other social locations (Singh et al., 2014), because gender affirmation is related to positive outcomes for individuals who may not fit into gender binaries (Goldenberg et al., 2019; Lelutiu-Weinberger et al., 2020). Additionally, parents' efficacy to effectively support their children has been associated with parents' gender diversity education, parental support systems (e.g., peers, providers), and time to integrate and adapt (Pullen Sansfaçon et al., 2020). Conclusively, affirmative family experiences for queer and 2STNB folx can be facilitated by effective and intentional professionals, supportive communities, and family openness and willingness to learn more and engage in advocacy (Chan, 2018; Katz-Wise et al., 2020; Roe, 2017; Salerno et al., 2022).

1.9 Implications for Practice and Policy

At the time of this writing, a wave of anti-queer and 2STNB legislation – mostly aimed at LGBTQ+ youth and young adults – has continued to sweep the United States. From bills that restrict 2STNB individuals from engaging in sports that align with their gender identity, to legislation purporting that helping 2STNB youth and young adults get access to gender affirming medical care is child abuse, to pushes for the use of "religious freedom" to allow healthcare providers to discriminate against LGBTQ+ individuals, LGBTQ+ communities are under attack (ACLU,

2022; Chappell, 2022). To be clear, assaults against LGBTQ+ individuals at the policy level are nothing new. However, as the societal visibility of LGBTQ+ identities and experiences increases, LGBTQ+ individuals' fears regarding backlash and increased discrimination are founded (Bockting et al., 2020). As we discussed throughout this chapter, the path to liberation for all is tied to the liberation of queer and 2STNB communities (Singh, 2016). The Western notion of the gender binary and subsequent norms and values like heterosexism restrict and harm all people and are offshoots of a system that privileges a few, while harming the majority. In order for liberation and collective healing to occur, we must engage in deep transformation at the sociopolitical level (Singh, 2020).

BIPOC queer and 2STNB people have paved the road for liberation, working in abolitionist movements to dismantle major carceral systems (e.g., Solutions Not Punishments in Atlanta; Bervera, 2019), create sustainable housing initiatives (e.g., House of Tulip in New Orleans; Clapp, 2021), and engage in advocacy and outreach efforts that change lives (e.g., TransLatin@ Coalition in Los Angeles; Ferrannini, 2021). For those of us in positions of power and privilege, we must link arms with such powerful BIPOC queer and 2STNB-led community-based organizations with our money, time, and other resources to support their missions. The creation of sustainable, long-term partnerships with BIPOC queer and 2STNB-led organizations is imperative in order to leverage power and amplify the knowledge, creativity, and resistance of community leadership. From engaging in street activism, lobbying state legislative bodies, using our vote to elevate those best positioned to make change, to getting involved in school parent-teacher associations and school district meetings, we all can leverage our awareness, knowledge, skills, and privilege to help make our society a more liberatory one with ready access to resources and opportunities to support the well-being of queer and 2STNB communities.

It is clear that our helping professions require deep transformation at the education, skill development, and theory implementation levels. Contemporary health, development, education, counseling, and psychology theory and practice are rooted in ways of knowing and healing from white, western epistemologies that are not always conducive to the work required for LGBTQ+ liberation. As previously reviewed, helping professionals should extend our work beyond the awareness, knowledge, and skills framework of cultural competence to deepen our personal understandings and relationships to gender and sexuality. Asking ourselves questions like "What did I learn about gender and sexuality in my personal upbringing?" or "How am I personally affected by cisnormativity and heterosexism?" can help us connect on a personal transformational level instead of staying at what Singh (2016) terms the "awareness" level of allyship (p. 756). We need to interrogate what we learned or did not learn in our training programs regarding gender and sexuality. Here, reflecting on questions like "What beliefs about gender and sexuality are embedded in my theoretical orientation or philosophy of helping?" and "What do I believe my role is in the fight for LGBTQ+ liberation and healing?" can be helpful. Additionally, teaching ourselves about the history of 2STNB and queer communities that have existed across time, culture, and continent (Stryker, 2017), and the role of European colonization in forming today's manifestation of cis/heteronormativity are ways we can recover historical memory conducive to our own healing, as well as helping the LGBTQ+ community heal (Singh, 2016). Understanding the ways the cisnormativity and heteronormativity pervade the helping professions theory and praxis, forming partnerships with 2STNB and queer communities to best understand the community's unique needs and strengths, tailoring approaches to be culturally responsive to unique understandings and relationships with gender and sexuality based in cultural and tradition, and stepping outside of the therapy room and into activism and advocacy roles are some ways practitioners can work toward liberation and collective healing (Chang & Singh, 2018; Singh, 2016; Singh & Dickey, 2017).

Questions for Thought and Discussion

1. What is the difference between affirmative and liberatory practice with queer and 2STNB clients?
2. How do intersectional inequities (e.g., heterosexism, sexism, racism) and other oppressions (e.g., ableism, classism, xenoprejudice) show up in helping professions training, practice, and research with queer and 2STNB people?
3. Why is resilience and important construct to understand in liberatory approaches with queer and 2STNB people?
4. What are the major domains of multicultural and social justice helping work with queer and 2STNB people?
5. What is your advocate role as a professional in practice with queer and 2STNB people?

Conflict of Interest We have no known conflict of interest to disclose

References

Abreu, R. L., & Gonzalez, K. A. (2020). Redefining collectivism: Family and community among sexual and gender diverse people of color and indigenous people: Introduction to the special issue. *Journal of GLBT Family Studies, 16*(2), 107–110. https://doi.org/10.1080/1550428X.2020.1736038

Abreu, R. L., Gonzalez, K. A., Capielo Rosario, C. C., Lindley, L., & Lockett, G. M. (2021a). "What American dream is this?": The effect of Trump's presidency on immigrant Latinx transgender people. *Journal of Counseling Psychology, 68*(6), 657–669. https://doi.org/10.1037/cou0000541

Abreu, R. L., Gonzalez, K. A., Capielo Rosario, C., Lockett, G. M., Lindley, L., & Lane, S. (2021b). "We are our own community": Immigrant Latinx transgender people community experiences. *Journal of Counseling Psychology, 68*(4), 390–403. https://doi.org/10.1037/cou0000546

Abreu, R. L., Sostre, J. P., Gonzalez, K. A., Lockett, G. M., & Matsuno, E. (2021c). "I am afraid for those kids who might find death preferable": Parental figures' reactions and coping strategies to bans on gender affirming care for transgender and gender diverse youth. *Psychology of Sexual Orientation and Gender Diversity., 9*, 500. https://doi.org/10.1037/sgd0000495

Abreu, R. L., Sostre, J. P., Gonzalez, K. A., Lockett, G. M., Matsuno, E., & Mosley, D. V. (2022). Impact of gender-affirming care bans on transgender and gender diverse youth: Parental figures' perspective. *Journal of Family Psychology, 36*(5), 643. https://doi.org/10.1037/fam0000987

Adames, H. Y., Chavez-Dueñas, N. Y., Sharma, S., & la Roche, M. J. (2018). Intersectionality in psychotherapy: The experiences of an AfroLatinx queer immigrant. *Psychotherapy, 55*(1), 73–79. https://doi.org/10.1037/pst0000152

Almeida, J., Johnson, R. M., Corliss, H. L., Molnar, B. E., & Azrael, D. (2009). Emotional distress among LGBT youth: The influence of perceived discrimination based on sexual orientation. *Journal of Youth and Adolescence, 38*(7), 1001–1014. https://doi.org/10.1007/s10964-009-9397-9

American Civil Liberties Union. (2022, May 20). *Legislation affecting LGBTQ rights across the country.* https://www.aclu.org/legislation-affecting-lgbtq-rights-across-country

American Counseling Association. (2010). Competencies for counseling with transgender clients. *Journal of LGBT Issues in Counseling, 4*(3–4), 135–159. https://doi.org/10.1080/15538605.2010.524839

American Counseling Association. (2014). *ACA code of ethics.* https://www.counseling.org/docs/default-source/default-document-library/2014-code-of-ethics-finaladdress.pdf

American Counseling Association. (2018). *ACA Advocacy Competencies.* https://www.counseling.org/docs/default-source/competencies/aca-advocacy-competencies-updated-may-2020.pdf?sfvrsn=f410212c_4

American Psychological Association. (2012). Guidelines for psychological practice with lesbian, gay and bisexual clients. *American Psychologist, 67*(1), 10–42. https://doi.org/10.1037/a0024659

American Psychological Association. (2015). Guidelines for psychological practice with transgender and gender nonconforming people. *American Psychologist, 70*(9), 832–864. https://doi.org/10.1037/a0039906

Anderson, A. D., Irwin, J. A., Brown, A. M., & Grala, C. L. (2020). "Your picture looks the same as my picture": An examination of passing in transgender communities. *Gender Issues, 37*(1), 44–60. https://doi.org/10.1007/s12147-019-09239-x

Andrzewjewski, J., Pampati, S., Steiner, R. J., Boyce, L., & Johns, M. M. (2020). Perspectives of transgender youth on parental support: Qualitative findings from the resilience and transgender youth study. *Health Education & Behavior, 48*(1), 74–81. https://doi.org/10.1177/1090198120965504

Asakura, K. (2017). Paving pathways through the pain: A grounded theory of resilience among lesbian, gay, bisexual, trans, and queer youth. *Journal of Research on Adolescence, 27*(3), 521–536. https://doi.org/10.1111/jora.12291

Asakura, K. (2019). Extraordinary acts to "show up": Conceptualizing resilience of LGBTQ youth. *Youth & Society, 51*(2), 268–285. https://doi.org/10.1177/0044118X16671430

Baams, L., Wilson, B. D., & Russell, S. T. (2019). LGBTQ youth in unstable housing and foster care. *Pediatrics, 143*(3), e20174211. https://doi.org/10.1542/peds.2017-4211

Bain, C. L., Grzanka, P. R., & Crowe, B. J. (2016). Toward a queer music therapy: The implications of queer theory for radically inclusive music therapy. *Arts in Psychotherapy, 50*, 22–33. https://doi.org/10.1016/j.aip.2016.03.004

Ball, T. C., Molina, L. E., & Branscombe, N. R. (2021). Consequences of interminority ingroup rejection for group identification and well-being. *Cultural Diversity and Ethnic Minority Psychology.* Advance online publication. https://doi.org/10.1037/cdp0000380.

Baker Miller, J. (1986). Toward a new psychology of women. Beacon Press.

Barr, S. M., Snyder, K. E., Adelson, J. L., & Budge, S. L. (2021). Posttraumatic stress in the trans community: The roles of anti-transgender bias, non-affirmation, and internalized transphobia. *Psychology of Sexual Orientation and Gender Diversity, 9*(40), 410–421. https://doi.org/10.1037/sgd0000500

Bervera, X. (2019, October 22). How an alliance of formerly incarcerated women, trans and queer leaders, and immigrant justice organizers closed down an Atlanta jail. *Medium.* https://medium.com/@xochitlrjac/how-an-alliance-of-formerly-incarcerated-women-trans-and-queer-leaders-and-immigrant-justice-6bf8ac2d8429

Bettergarcia, J., Matsuno, E., & Conover, K. J. (2021). Training mental health providers in queer-affirming care: A systematic review. *Psychology of Sexual Orientation and Gender Diversity, 8*(3), 365–377. https://doi.org/10.1037/sgd0000514

Bockting, W., Barucco, R., LeBlanc, A., Singh, A., Mellman, W., Dolezal, C., & Ehrhardt, A. (2020). Sociopolitical change and transgender people's perceptions of vulnerability and resilience. *Sexuality Research and Social Policy, 17*(1), 162–174. https://doi.org/10.1007/s13178-019-00381-5

Brooks, V. R. (1981). *Minority stress and lesbian women*. Lexington Books.

Brown, C., & Keller, C. J. (2018). The 2016 presidential election outcome: Fears, tension, and resiliency of GLBTQ communities. *Journal of GLBT Family Studies, 14*(1–2), 101–129. https://doi.org/10.1080/1550428X.2017.1420847

Budge, S. L., Rossman, H. K., & Howard, K. A. S. (2014). Coping and psychological distress among genderqueer individuals: The moderating effect of social support. *Journal of LGBT Issues in Counseling, 8*(1), 95–117. https://doi.org/10.1080/15538605.2014.853641

Casanova-Perez, R., Apodaca, C., Bascom, E., Mohanraj, D., Lane, C., Vidyarthi, D., … & Hartzler, A. L. (2021). Broken down by bias: Healthcare biases experienced by BIPOC and LGBTQ+ patients. In *AMIA annual symposium proceedings*: *Vol. 2021* (p. 275). American Medical Informatics Association.

Cerezo, A., Morales, A., Quintero, D., & Rothman, S. (2014). Trans migrations: Exploring life at the intersection of transgender identity and immigration. *Psychology of Sexual Orientation and Gender Diversity, 1*(2), 170–180. https://doi.org/10.1037/sgd0000031

Chan, C. D. (2018). Families as transformative allies to trans youth of color: Positioning intersectionality as analysis to demarginalize political systems of oppression. *Journal of GLBT Family Studies, 14*(1–2), 43–60. https://doi.org/10.1080/1550428X.2017.1421336

Chan, C. D., Frank, C. D., DeMeyer, M., Joshi, A., Andrade Vargas, E., & Silverio, N. (2021). Counseling older LGBTQ+ adults of color: Relational-cultural theory in practice. *The Professional Counselor, 11*(3), 370–382. https://doi.org/10.15241/cdc.11.3.370

Chaney, M. P., & Whitman, J. S. (2020). Affirmative wellness counseling with older LGBTQ+ adults. *Journal of Mental Health Counseling, 42*(4), 303–322. https://doi.org/10.17744/mehc.42.4.02

Chang, S. C., & Singh, A. A. (2018). *A clinician's guide to gender-affirming care: Working with transgender and gender nonconforming clients*. New Harbinger Publications.

Chappell, B. (2022, May 13). *Texas Supreme Court oks state child abuse inquiries into the families of trans kids*. Special series: Efforts to restrict rights for LGBTQ youth. https://www.npr.org/2022/05/13/1098779201/texas-supreme-court-transgender-gender-affirming-child-abuse

Clapp, J. (2021, May 31). A long time coming: House of Tulip puts trans and gender-nonconforming New Orleanians in control of their housing. *Gambit*. https://www.nola.com/gambit/news/the_latest/article_59d5a2c4-bf26-11eb-a463-6b340d8a4c1a.html

Comstock, D. L., Hammer, T. R., Strentzsch, J., Cannon, K., Parsons, J., & Ii, G. S. (2008). Relational-cultural theory: A framework for bridging relational, multicultural, and social justice competencies. *Journal of Counseling & Development, 86*, 279–287. https://doi.org/10.1002/j.1556-6678.2008.tb00510.x

Coulter, R. W., Birkett, M., Corliss, H. L., Hatzenbuehler, M. L., Mustanski, B., & Stall, R. D. (2016). Associations between LGBTQ-affirmative school climate and adolescent drinking behaviors. *Drug and Alcohol Dependence, 161*, 340–347. https://doi.org/10.1016/j.drugalcdep.2016.02.022

Council for Accreditation of Counseling & Related Educational Programs. (2016). 2016 CACREP Standards. Retrieved from http://www.cacrep.org/wp-content/uploads/2017/08/2016-Standards-with-citations.pdf

Counselors for Social Justice (CSJ) Ethics Committee. (2011). The counselors for social justice (CSJ) code of ethics. *Journal for Social Action in Counseling and Psychology, 3*, 1–21.

Craig, S. L., McInroy, L., McCready, L. T., & Alaggia, R. (2015). Media: A catalyst for resilience in lesbian, gay, bisexual, transgender, and queer youth. *Journal of LGBT Youth, 12*(3), 254–275. https://doi.org/10.1080/19361653.2015.1040193

Crenshaw, K. (1989). Demarginalizing the intersection of race and sex: A black feminist critique of antidiscrimination doctrine, feminist theory and antiracist politics. *University of Chicago Legal Forum, 1989*(1), 139. https://doi.org/10.4324/9780429499142-5

Day, J. K., Fish, J. N., Grossman, A. H., & Russell, S. T. (2020). Gay-straight alliances, inclusive policy, and school climate: LGBTQ youths' experiences of social support and bullying. *Journal of Research on Adolescence, 30*(S2), 418–430. https://doi.org/10.1111/jora.12487

DePedro, T. K., Jackson, C., Campbell, E., Gilley, J., & Ciarelli, B. (2016). Creating trans-inclusive schools: Introductory activities that enhance the critical consciousness of future educators. *International Journal of Teaching and Learning in Higher Education, 28*(2), 293–301.

Drapela, V. J. (1990). The value of theories for counseling practitioners. *International Journal for the Advancement of Counselling, 13*, 19–26. https://doi.org/10.1007/BF00154639

Drazdowski, T. K., Perrin, P. B., Trujillo, M., Sutter, M., Benotsch, E. G., & Snipes, D. J. (2016). Structural equation modeling of the effects of racism, LGBTQ discrimination, and internalized oppression on illicit drug use in LGBTQ people of color. *Drug and Alcohol Dependence, 159*, 255–262. https://doi.org/10.1016/j.drugalcdep.2015.12.029

Eccles, J. S., & Roeser, R. W. (2011). Schools as developmental contexts during adolescence. *Journal of Research on Adolescence, 21*(1), 225–241. https://doi.org/10.1111/j.1532-7795.2010.00725.x

Estevez, R. (2022). *Talk about resilient – We just don't give up: The risk and resilience experiences of the Latinx trans and nonbinary community*. [Doctoral dissertation, University of Georgia]. ProQuest Dissertations & Theses Global.

Ferrannini, J. (2021, April 21). *New TGI-led alliance seeks $15 million for state trans health fund.* Bay Area Reporter. https://www.ebar.com/news/latest_news//304196

Fitzgerald, K. J. (2017). Understanding racialized homophobic and transphobic violence. In S. Weissinger, D. Mack, & E. Elwood (Eds.), *Violence against black bodies* (pp. 53–70). Routledge.

Flaskerud, J. H., & Lesser, J. (2018). The current socio-political climate and psychological distress among transgender people. *Issues in Mental Health Nursing, 39*(1), 93–96. https://doi.org/10.1080/01612840.2017.1368751

Flores, C. A., & Sheely-Moore, A. I. (2020). Relational-cultural theory–based interventions with LGBTQ college students. *Journal of College Counseling, 23*(1), 71–84. https://doi.org/10.1002/jocc.12150

Follins, L. D., Walker, J. N. J., & Lewis, M. K. (2014). Resilience in black lesbian, gay, bisexual, and transgender individuals: A critical review of the literature. *Journal of Gay & Lesbian Mental Health, 18*(2), 190–212. https://doi.org/10.1080/19359705.2013.828343

Frost, D. M., Fine, M., Torre, M. E., & Cabana, A. (2019). Minority stress, activism, and health in the context of economic precarity: Results from a national participatory action survey of lesbian, gay, bisexual, transgender, queer, and gender non-conforming youth. *American Journal of Community Psychology, 63*(3–4), 511–526. https://doi.org/10.1002/ajcp.12326

García, J. J., & Kijak, M. (2021). Cerebrovascular disease risk factor burden in LGBTQ PoC. In J. García (Ed.), *Heart, brain and mental health disparities for LGBTQ people of color* (pp. 81–92). Palgrave Macmillan. https://doi.org/10.1007/978-3-030-70060-7

García, J. J., & Serpas, D. G. (2021). Cardiovascular disease risk factor burden in LGBTQ PoC. In J. García (Ed.), *Heart, brain and mental health disparities for LGBTQ people of color* (pp. 55–67). Palgrave Macmillan. https://doi.org/10.1007/978-3-030-70060-7

Ghabrial, M. A. (2017). "Trying to figure out where we belong": Narratives of racialized sexual minorities on community, identity, discrimination, and health. *Sexuality Research and Social Policy, 14*(1), 42–55. https://doi.org/10.1007/s13178-016-0229-x

Goldberg, A. E., Beemyn, G., & Smith, J. A. Z. (2019). What is needed, what is valued: Trans students' perspectives on trans-inclusive policies and practices in higher education. *Journal of*

Educational and Psychological Consultation, 29(1), 27–67. https://doi.org/10.1080/10474412.2018.1480376

Goldenberg, T., Jadwin-Cakmak, L., Popoff, E., Reisner, S. L., Campbell, B. A., & Harper, G. W. (2019). Stigma, gender affirmation, and primary healthcare use among black transgender youth. *Journal of Adolescent Health, 65*(4), 483–490. https://doi.org/10.1016/j.jadohealth.2019.04.029

Goldenberg, T., Gamarel, K. E., Reisner, S. L., Jadwin-Cakmak, L., & Harper, G. W. (2021). Gender affirmation as a source of resilience for addressing stigmatizing healthcare experiences of transgender youth of color. *Annals of Behavioral Medicine, 55*(12), 1168–1183. https://doi.org/10.1093/abm/kaab011

Gonzalez, K. A., Abreu, R. L., Arora, S., Lockett, G. M., & Sostre, J. (2021). "Previous resilience has taught me that I can survive anything:" LGBTQ resilience during the COVID-19 pandemic. *Psychology of Sexual Orientation and Gender Diversity, 8*(2), 133–144. https://doi.org/10.1037/sgd0000501

González-Álvarez, R., Brummelaar, M. T., Orwa, S., & López López, M. (2022). 'I actually know that things will get better': The many pathways to resilience of LGBTQIA+ youth in out-of-home care. *Children & Society, 36*(2), 234–248. https://doi.org/10.1111/chso.12464

Gorman, K. R., Shipherd, J. C., Collins, K. M., Gunn, H. A., Rubin, R. O., Rood, B. A., & Pantalone, D. W. (2020). Coping, resilience, and social support among transgender and gender diverse individuals experiencing gender-related stress. *Psychology of Sexual Orientation and Gender Diversity, 9*(1), 37. https://doi.org/10.1037/sgd0000455

Green, A. E., Price, M. N., & Dorison, S. H. (2022). Cumulative minority stress and suicide risk among LGBTQ youth. *American Journal of Community Psychology, 69*(1–2), 157–168. https://doi.org/10.1002/ajcp.12553

Hailey, J., Burton, W., & Arscott, J. (2020). We are family: Chosen and created families as a protective factor against racialized trauma and anti-LGBTQ oppression among African American sexual and gender minority youth. *Journal of GLBT Family Studies, 16*(2), 176–191. https://doi.org/10.1080/1550428X.2020.1724133

Harper, A., Finnerty, P., Martinez, M., Brace, A., Crethar, H. C., Loos, B., Harper, B., Graham, S., Singh, A., Kocet, M., Travis, L., Lambert, S., Burnes, T., Dickey, L. M., & Hammer, T. R. (2013). Association for lesbian, gay, bisexual, and transgender issues in counseling competencies for counseling with lesbian, gay, bisexual, queer, questioning, intersex, and ally individuals. *Journal of LGBT Issues in Counseling, 7*(1), 2–43. https://doi.org/10.1080/15538605.2013.755444

Hillier, A., Kroehle, K., Edwards, H., & Graves, G. (2020). Risk, resilience, resistance and situated agency of trans high school students. *Journal of LGBT Youth, 17*(4), 384–407. https://doi.org/10.1080/19361653.2019.1668326

Horne, S. G., McGinley, M., Yel, N., & Maroney, M. R. (2022). The stench of bathroom bills and anti-transgender legislation: Anxiety and depression among transgender, nonbinary, and cisgender LGBQ people during a state referendum. *Journal of Counseling Psychology, 69*(1), 1–13. https://doi.org/10.1037/cou0000558

Hudson, K. D., & Romanelli, M. (2020). "We are powerful people": Health-promoting strengths of LGBTQ communities of color. *Qualitative Health Research, 30*(8), 1156–1170. https://doi.org/10.1177/1049732319837572

Hull, K. E., & Ortyl, T. A. (2019). Conventional and cutting-edge: Definitions of family in LGBT communities. *Sexuality Research and Social Policy, 16*(1), 31–43. https://doi.org/10.1007/s13178-018-0324-2

James, S. E., Herman, J. L., Rankin, S., Keisling, M., Mottet, L., & Anafi, M. (2016). *Executive summary of the report of the 2015 U.S. transgender survey*. National Center for Transgender Equality.

Johns, M. M., Lowry, R., Haderxhanaj, L. T., Rasberry, C. N., Robin, L., Scales, L., et al. (2020). Trends in violence victimization and suicide risk by sexual identity among high school students – Youth risk behavior survey, United States, 2015–2019. *MMWR supplements, 69*(1), 19–27.

Jordan, J. V. (2001). A relational-cultural model: Healing through mutual empathy. *Bulletin of the Menninger Clinic, 65*, 92–103. https://doi.org/10.1521/bumc.65.1.92.18707

Jordan, J. V. (2008). Learning at the margin: New models of strength. *Women & Therapy, 31*(2–4), 189–208. https://doi.org/10.1080/02703140802146365

Katz-Wise, S. L., Godwin, E. G., Parsa, N., Brown, C. A., Sansfaçon, A. P., Goldman, R., MacNish, M., Rosal, M. C., & Austin, S. B. (2020). Using family and ecological systems approaches to conceptualize family and community-based experiences of transgender and/or nonbinary youth from the trans teen and family narratives project. *Psychology of Sexual Orientation and Gender Diversity, 9*(1), 21–36. https://doi.org/10.1037/sgd0000442

Knutson, D., Matsuno, E., Goldbach, C., Hashtpari, H., & Smith, N. G. (2022). Advocating for transgender and nonbinary affirmative spaces in graduate education. *Higher Education, 83*(2), 461–479. https://doi.org/10.1007/s10734-020-00673-5

Koech, J. M., Sostre, J. P., Lockett, G. M., Gonzalez, K. A., & Abreu, R. L. (2022). Resisting by existing: Trans Latinx mental health, well-being, and resilience in the United States. In R. Chaparro & M. Prado (Eds.), *Latinx queer psychology* (pp. 43–67). Springer. https://doi.org/10.1007/978-3-030-82250-7

Lardier, D. T., Pinto, S. A., Brammer, M. K., Garcia-Reid, P., & Reid, R. J. (2020). The relationship between queer identity, social connection, school bullying, and suicidal ideations among youth of color. *Journal of LGBT Issues in Counseling, 14*(2), 74–99. https://doi.org/10.1080/15538605.2020.1753623

Layland, E. K., Exten, C., Mallory, A. B., Williams, N. D., & Fish, J. N. (2020). Suicide attempt rates and associations with discrimination are greatest in early adulthood for sexual minority adults across diverse racial and ethnic groups, *LGBT Health, 7*(8), 439–447.

Leland, W., & Stockwell, A. (2019). A self-assessment tool for cultivating affirming practices with transgender and gender-nonconforming (TGNC) clients, supervisees, students, and colleagues. *Behavior Analysis in Practice, 12*(4), 816–825. https://doi.org/10.1007/s40617-019-00375-0

Lelutiu-Weinberger, C., English, D., & Sandanapitchai, P. (2020). The roles of gender affirmation and discrimination in the resilience of transgender individuals in the US. *Behavioral Medicine, 46*(3–4), 175–188. https://doi.org/10.1080/08964289.2020.1725414

Lelutiu-Weinberger, C., Clark, K. A., & Pachankis, J. E. (2022). Mental health provider training to improve LGBTQ competence and reduce implicit and explicit bias: A randomized controlled trial of online and in-person delivery. *Psychology of Sexual Orientation and Gender Diversity*. Advance online publication. https://doi.org/10.1037/sgd0000560.

Levin, N. J., Kattari, S. K., Piellusch, E. K., & Watson, E. (2020). "We just take care of each other": Navigating 'chosen family' in the context of health, illness, and the mutual provision of care amongst queer and transgender young adults. *International Journal of Environmental Research and Public Health, 17*(19), 1–20. https://doi.org/10.3390/ijerph17197346

Lockett, G. M., Brooks, J. E., Abreu, R. L., & Sostre, J. P. (2022). "I want to go to a place that's openly talking about the experiences of people of color who also identify as LGBTQ+": Cultural, religious, and spiritual experiences of LGBTQ people of color. *Spirituality in Clinical Practice*. Advance online publication. https://doi.org/10.1037/scp0000288.

Mahowald, L. (2021). *LGBT people of color enouchter heightened discrimination: 2020 survey results on experiences in health care, housing, and education.* The Center for American Progress. https://www.americanprogress.org/article/lgbtq-people-color-encounter-heightened-discrimination/

Mallory, A. B., & Russell, S. T. (2021). Intersections of racial discrimination and LGB victimization for mental health: A prospective study of sexual minority youth of color. *Journal of Youth and Adolescence, 50*(7), 1353–1368. https://doi.org/10.1007/s10964-021-01443-x

Matsuno, E. (2019). Nonbinary-affirming psychological interventions. *Cognitive and Behavioral Practice, 26*(4), 617–628. https://doi.org/10.1016/j.cbpra.2018.09.003

McBride, R. S. (2021). A literature review of the secondary school experiences of trans youth. *Journal of LGBT Youth, 18*(2), 103–134. https://doi.org/10.1080/19361653.2020.1727815

McConnell, E. A., Janulis, P., Phillips, G., 2nd, Truong, R., & Birkett, M. (2018). Multiple minority stress and LGBT community resilience among sexual minority men. *Psychology of Sexual Orientation and Gender Diversity, 5*(1), 1–12. https://doi.org/10.1037/sgd0000265

McCullough, R., Dispenza, F., Parker, L. K., Viehl, C. J., Chang, C. Y., & Murphy, T. M. (2017). The counseling experiences of transgender and gender nonconforming clients. *Journal of Counseling and Development, 95*(4), 423–434. https://doi.org/10.1002/jcad.12157

Menakem, R. (2017). *My grandmother's hands: Racialized trauma and the pathway to mending our hearts and bodies*. Central Recovery Press.

Mereish, E. H. (2019). Substance use and misuse among sexual and gender minority youth. *Current Opinion in Psychology, 30*, 123–127. https://doi.org/10.1016/j.copsyc.2019.05.002

Meyer, I. H. (2015). Resilience in the study of minority stress and health of sexual and gender minorities. *Psychology of Sexual Orientation and Gender Diversity, 2*(3), 209–213. https://doi.org/10.1037/sgd0000132

Morton, M. H., Dworsky, A., Matjasko, J. L., Curry, S. R., Schlueter, D., Chávez, R., & Farrell, A. F. (2018). Prevalence and correlates of youth homelessness in the United States. *Journal of Adolescent Health, 62*(1), 14–21. https://doi.org/10.1016/j.jadohealth.2017.10.006

Mosley, D. V., Neville, H. A., Chavez-Dueñas, N. Y., Adames, H. Y., Lewis, J. A., & French, B. H. (2020). Radical hope in revolting times: Proposing a culturally relevant psychological framework. *Social and Personality Psychology Compass, 14*(1). https://doi.org/10.1111/spc3.12512

Mosley, D., McNeil-Young, V., Bridges, B., Adam, S., Colson, A., Crowley, M., & Lee, L. (2021). Toward radical healing: A qualitative metasynthesis exploring oppression and liberation among black queer people. *Psychology of Sexual Orientation and Gender Diversity, 8*(3), 292–313. https://doi.org/10.1037/sgd0000522

National Association of Social Workers [NASW]. (2015a). *Lesbian gay and bisexual issues*. In Social work speaks: National Association of Social Workers policy statements, 2015–2017 (10th ed., pp. 198–206). NASW Press.

National Association of Social Workers [NASW]. (2015b). *Transgender and gender identity issues*. In Social work speaks: National Association of Social Workers policy statements, 2015–2017 (10th ed., pp. 311–315). NASW Press.

National Organization of Human Services [NOHS]. (2015). *Ethical standards for human services professionals*. Retrieved from http://www.nationalhumanservices.org/ethical-standards-for-hs-professionals

Needham, B. L., & Austin, E. L. (2010). Sexual orientation, parental support, and health during the transition to young adulthood. *Journal of Youth and Adolescence, 39*(10), 1189–1198. https://doi.org/10.1007/s10964-010-9533-6

Noyola, N., Sánchez, M., & Cardemil, E. V. (2020). Minority stress and coping among sexual diverse Latinxs. *Journal of Latinx Psychology, 8*(1), 58–82. https://doi.org/10.1037/lat0000143

Parmenter, J. G., Galliher, R. V., Wong, E., & Perez, D. (2021). An intersectional approach to understanding LGBTQ+ people of color's access to LGBTQ+ community resilience. *Journal of Counseling Psychology, 68*(6), 629–641. https://doi.org/10.1037/cou0000578

Patton, J., & Reicherzer, S. (2010). Inviting "Kate's" authenticity: Relational cultural theory applied in work with a transsexual sex worker of color using the competencies for counseling with transgender clients. *Journal of LGBT Issues in Counseling, 4*(3), 214–227. https://doi.org/10.1080/15538605.2010.524846

Prilleltensky, I. (2003). Understanding, resisting, and overcoming oppression: Toward psychopolitical validity. *American Journal of Community Psychology, 31*(2), 195–201. https://doi.org/10.1023/a:1023043108210

Prilleltensky, I. (2008). The role of power in wellness, oppression, and liberation: The promise of psychopolitical validity. *Journal of Community Psychology, 36*(2), 116–136. https://doi.org/10.1002/jcop.20225

Pullen Sansfaçon, A., Kirichenko, V., Holmes, C., Feder, S., Lawson, M. L., Ghosh, S., Ducharme, J., Temple Newhook, J., & Suerich-Gulick, F. (2020). Parents' journeys to acceptance and support of gender-diverse and trans children and youth. *Journal of Family Issues, 41*(8), 1214–1236. https://doi.org/10.1177/0192513X19888779

Ratts, M. J., Singh, A. A., Nassar-Mcmillan, S., Butler, S. K., & McCullough, J. R. (2016). Multicultural and social justice counseling competencies: Guidelines for the counseling profession. *Journal of Multicultural Counseling and Development, 44*(1), 28–48. https://doi.org/10.1002/jmcd.12035

Robinson, B. A. (2018). Conditional families and lesbian, gay, bisexual, transgender, and queer youth homelessness: Gender, sexuality, family instability, and rejection. *Journal of Marriage and Family, 80*(2), 383–396. https://doi.org/10.1111/jomf.12466

Robinson, B. A. (2020). The lavender scare in homonormative times: Policing, hyper-incarceration, and LGBTQ youth homelessness. *Gender & Society, 34*(2), 210–232. https://doi.org/10.1177/0891243220906172

Roe, S. (2017). "Family support would have been like amazing" LGBTQ youth experiences with parental and family support. *The Family Journal, 25*(1), 55–62. https://doi.org/10.1177/1066480716679651

Russell, S. T., Ryan, C., Russell Toomey, A. B., Rafael Diaz, M. M., & Jorge Sanchez, M. (2011). Lesbian, gay, bisexual, and transgender adolescent xchool victimization: Implications for young adult health and adjustment. *The Journal of School Health, 81*(5), 223–230. https://doi.org/10.1111/j.1746-1561.2011.00583.x

Salerno, J. P., Gattamorta, K. A., & Williams, N. D. (2022). Impact of family rejection and racism on sexual and gender minority stress among LGBTQ young people of color during COVID-19. *Psychological Trauma: Theory, Research, Practice, and Policy*. Advance online publication. https://doi.org/10.1037/tra0001254.

Schmitz, R. M., & Tyler, K. A. (2019). 'Life has actually become more clear': An examination of resilience among LGBTQ young adults. *Sexualities, 22*(4), 710–733. https://doi.org/10.1177/1363460718770451

Schmitz, R. M., Robinson, B. A., & Sanchez, J. (2020a). Intersectional family systems approach: LGBTQ+ Latino/a youth, family dynamics, and stressors. *Family Relations, 69*(4), 832–848. https://doi.org/10.1111/fare.12448

Schmitz, R. M., Robinson, B. A., Tabler, J., Welch, B., & Rafaqut, S. (2020b). LGBTQ+ Latino/a young people's interpretations of stigma and mental health: An intersectional minority stress perspective. *Society and Mental Health, 10*(2), 163–179. https://doi.org/10.1177/2156869319847248

Singh, A. A. (2013). Transgender youth of color and resilience: Negotiating oppression and finding support. *Sex Roles, 68*(11–12), 690–702. https://doi.org/10.1007/s11199-012-0149-z

Singh, A. A. (2016). Moving from affirmation to liberation in psychological practice with transgender and gender nonconforming clients. *American Psychologist, 71*(8), 755–762. https://doi.org/10.1037/amp0000106

Singh, A. A. (2017). Understanding trauma and supporting resilience with LGBT people of color. In K. L. Eckstrand & J. E. Potter (Eds.), *Trauma, resilience, and health promotion in LGBT patients* (pp. 113–119). Springer.

Singh, A. (2020). Building a counseling psychology of liberation: The path behind us, under us, and before us. *The Counseling Psychologist, 28*(8), 1109–1130. https://doi.org/10.1177/0011000020959007

Singh, A., & Dickey, L. M. (Eds.). (2017). *Affirmative counseling and psychological practice with transgender and gender nonconforming clients.* American Psychological Association. https://doi.org/10.1037/14957-000.

Singh, A. A., & McKleroy, V. S. (2011). "Just getting out of bed is a revolutionary act": The resilience of transgender people of color who have survived traumatic life events. *Traumatology, 17*(2), 34–44. https://doi.org/10.1177/1534765610369261

Singh, A. A., & Moss, L. (2016). Using relational-cultural theory in LGBTQQ counseling: Addressing heterosexism and enhancing relational competencies. *Journal of Counseling and Development, 94*(4), 398–404. https://doi.org/10.1002/jcad.12098

Singh, A. A., Hays, D. G., & Watson, L. S. (2011). Strength in the face of adversity: Resilience strategies of transgender individuals. *Journal of Counseling & Development, 89*(1), 20–27. https://doi.org/10.1002/j.1556-6678.2011.tb00057.x

Singh, A. A., Meng, S. E., & Hansen, A. W. (2014). "I am my own gender": Resilience strategies of trans youth. *Journal of Counseling and Development, 92*(2), 208–218. https://doi.org/10.1002/j.1556-6676.2014.00150.x

Singh, A. A., Appling, B., & Trepal, H. (2020a). Using the multicultural and social justice counseling competencies to decolonize counseling practice: The important roles of theory, power, and action. *Journal of Counseling and Development, 98*(3), 261–271. https://doi.org/10.1002/jcad.12321

Singh, A. A., Parker, B., Aqil, A. R., & Thacker, F. (2020b). Liberation psychology and LGBTQ+ communities: Naming colonization, uplifting resilience, and reclaiming ancient his-stories, her-stories, and t-stories. In L. Comas-Díaz & E. Torres Rivera (Eds.), *Liberation psychology: Theory, method, practice, and social justice* (pp. 207–224). American Psychological Association. https://doi.org/10.1037/0000198-012

Snapp, S. D., Hoenig, J. M., Fields, A., & Russell, S. T. (2015). Messy, butch, and queer: LGBTQ youth and the school-to-prison pipeline. *Journal of Adolescent Research, 30*(1), 57–82. https://doi.org/10.1177/0743558414557625

Stone, A. L., Nimmons, E. A., Salcido, R., Jr., & Schnarrs, P. W. (2020). Multiplicity, race, and resilience: Transgender and non-binary people building community. *Sociological Inquiry, 90*(2), 226–248. https://doi.org/10.1111/soin.12341

Stryker, S. (2017). *Transgender history: The roots of today's revolution*. Hachette.

Sutter, M., & Perrin, P. B. (2016). Discrimination, mental health, and suicidal ideation among LGBTQ people of color. *Journal of Counseling Psychology, 63*(1), 98–105. https://doi.org/10.1037/cou0000126

Taliaferro, L. A., & Muehlenkamp, J. J. (2017). Nonsuicidal self-injury and suicidality among sexual minority youth: Risk factors and protective connectedness factors. *Academic Pediatrics, 17*(7), 715–722. https://doi.org/10.1016/j.acap.2016.11.002

Toomey, R. B., Huynh, V. W., Jones, S. K., Lee, S., & Revels-Macalinao, M. (2017). Sexual minority youth of color: A content analysis and critical review of the literature. *Journal of Gay and Lesbian Mental Health, 21*(1), 3–31. https://doi.org/10.1080/19359705.2016.1217499

Travers, A., Marchbank, J., Boulay, N., Jordan, S., & Reed, K. (2022). Talking back: Trans youth and resilience in action. *Journal of LGBT Youth, 19*(1), 1–30. https://doi.org/10.1080/19361653.2020.1758275

Vanderwaal, C. J., Sedlacek, D., & Lane, L. (2017). The impact of family rejection or acceptance among LGBT+ millennials in the seventh-day Adventist church. *Journal of the North American Association of Christians in Social Work, 44*(1 & 2), 72–95.

Velez, B. L., Moradi, B., & DeBlaere, C. (2015). Multiple oppressions and the mental health of sexual minority Latina/o individuals. *The Counseling Psychologist, 43*(1), 7–38. https://doi.org/10.1177/0011000014542836

White Hughto, J. M., Reisner, S. L., & Pachankis, J. E. (2015). Transgender stigma and health: A critical review of stigma determinants, mechanisms, and interventions. *Social Science and Medicine, 147*, 222–231. https://doi.org/10.1016/j.socscimed.2015.11.010

Yadegarfard, M., Meinhold-Bergmann, M. E., & Ho, R. (2014). Family rejection, social isolation, and loneliness as predictors of negative health outcomes (depression, suicidal ideation, and sexual risk behavior) among Thai male-to-female transgender adolescents. *Journal of LGBT Youth, 11*(4), 347–363. https://doi.org/10.1080/19361653.2014.910483

Chapter 2
Families of Transgender and Gender Expansive Persons: Support, Acceptance, Resilience, and Advocacy

Alfred F. Carlozzi

2.1 Introduction

It is important at the onset to acknowledge the social and political context in which this discussion of families of transgender and gender diverse persons is taking place. Helping professionals (social workers, child development professionals, educators, counselors, psychologists, and others) have garnered much knowledge and understanding of transgender and gender diverse persons, and there have been significant advances in the development of best practices for treating this population and their families. There have also been meaningful gains in protecting the civil rights of transgender and gender diverse persons, including institutional policies, federal guidance, and several court cases (Bryant & Young, 2019). We are also living in a time of extreme backlash against these gains that have been made, primarily at the state level, with one state even going so far as to criminalize parents who pursue affirmative health care for their transgender children, encouraging citizens to report such supportive parents as child abusers (New York Times, April 8, 2022). The ACLU and many professional and civil rights organizations have spoken out against such laws and policies that harm transgender persons and their families. Despite the progress made in understanding transgender and gender diverse persons, the battle to support them with what we know are best practices and the struggle to protect their civil rights continues in the culture war waged against them, their caregivers, and their service providers.

Most of what I have to share here is derived from several experiences, including the following: 1) serving for ten years as co-facilitator of a support group for parents of transgender and gender diverse youth at the Dennis R. Neill Equality Center in

A. F. Carlozzi (✉)
Oklahoma State University, Stillwater, OK, USA
e-mail: al.carlozzi@okstate.edu

J. M. Koch et al. (eds.), *Identity as Resilience in Minoritized Communities*, Emerging Issues in Family and Individual Resilience,
https://doi.org/10.1007/978-3-031-38977-1_2

Tulsa, Oklahoma; 2) providing counseling services to transgender and gender diverse persons, their spouses, and their families in my private psychology practice and supervising the provision of such services by interns at the Al Carlozzi Center for Counseling at Oklahoma State University-Tulsa; and 3) reviewing what has been written about the experiences and treatment of transgender persons and their families in order to make meaningful contributions to the literature on how best to assist them. In past publications, I have used the term *gender diverse*, which I believe is a less potentially pejorative term than the terms *gender variant* or *gender nonconforming*. In this chapter, I use the term *gender expansive*, adopted by Keo-Meier and Ehrensaft (2018), to include all gender identities other than cisgender and binary transgender identities (such as gender nonbinary, gender fluid, agender, etc.). In other words, the term gender expansive includes gender identities beyond the male or female binary. This term seems both accurate and more positive than previously used terms. Given the experiences enumerated above, what I have learned and what I can offer to service providers, educators, and families who wish to be helpful to transgender and gender expansive persons is described in this chapter.

2.2 Families with Transgender and Gender Expansive Youth

Families vary in degree and pace of acceptance and affirmation of their transgender or gender expansive family member. When a child, teen, young adult, or adult comes out as transgender or gender expansive to their family, parents and other family members can find adapting to this change in their loved one challenging. Some accept and adapt quite readily and are not surprised by this declaration of their loved one's gender identity. Others seem to be shocked by the disclosure, and may experience considerable grief, anxiety, and worry about the health, well-being, and future of their loved one. Many parents of transgender youth, for example, work through the well-known stages of grief (Kubler-Ross, 1970). They may at first deny the reality confronting them, hoping that this is a phase their child is going through, and move at their own pace from denial to anger, bargaining, depression, and eventual acceptance (Carlozzi, 2019). Lev and Alie (2012) also delineated several common stages that parents work through in their journey from turmoil, stress, and conflict to eventual acceptance and support. As Ryan et al. (2010) have described the family's adjustment to children who come out as LGBTQ, parents of transgender and gender expansive youth may vacillate between being accepting and supportive some of the time and rejecting at other times, as they navigate through their own transition in the identity of their family. Unfortunately, there are some parents who remain fixed at the earliest of stages, never get to acceptance and support, and become verbally and/or physically abusive toward their transgender or gender expansive child (Grossman et al., 2011). This is particularly concerning in light of the finding from the U.S. Transgender Survey that family support is associated with positive outcomes for transgender youth, and family rejection is associated with negative outcomes, such as depression, suicidality, self-harm, and substance abuse (James et al., 2016).

It is important to note that a family member's change in gender identity can effect a change in the identity of the family itself, sending what some might experience as shock waves through the family that can affect relationships between family members. Parents may conflict about how best to respond, siblings may be supportive or non-supportive, and reactions of extended family members may also be a matter of considerable concern to some or all in the nuclear family. The age of a sibling when their sibling comes out as transgender or gender expansive matters (Ehrensaft, 2019; Kuvalanka et al., 2014). Pre-school age children seem to adapt more readily, and the attention, playfulness, and overall attachment to their sibling seems to matter more than seeming changes in their gender. Older, school-age children and teenage siblings may be more concerned about what others think, and experience greater loss, embarrassment, and anger that could take some time to work through (Ehrensaft, 2019). Kuvalanka et al. (2014) described how one teenager asked his transgender sibling to postpone transitioning until adulthood because doing so after the sibling left home would have less impact on this younger sibling's life. Eventually, after educating himself, this same sibling came around to become an ardent supporter and advocate for his new sister.

2.3 Extended Family

Worries about reactions of those outside of the nuclear family are also common, as parents and their children struggle with how and when to come out to others in the extended family, as well as teachers and others at school, religious, and other community contexts. Reactions of those outside of the nuclear family also vary (Carlozzi, 2019). Grandparents, aunts, uncles, and cousins may be immediately accepting, while others may not know how to respond at first, try their best to be kind and supportive, but need help understanding what is happening to their loved ones. Parents of transgender and gender expansive youth, who hopefully are further down the road of understanding and supportiveness, can provide educational resources that they have found to be helpful to extended family members. They can listen to their concerns and provide information and reassurance that their nuclear family is affirming, supportive, and resilient, and can handle this change in the family. Such a presentation of support and affirmation for their transgender or gender expansive child, teen, or young adult, can strengthen the family's resilience and resolve to advocate for their child's rights and well-being (Carlozzi, 2019).

There are some extended family members who are outright resistant and refuse to accept their transgender or gender expansive family member and who condemn the parents for their acceptance and affirmation. Facing such resistance can also strengthen the nuclear family's resolve to act in the best interests of their child. I know of one mother who told her religiously conservative extended family at a family gathering in her home that her child is transgender, that this is her new name, that he is now she, and if anyone in the room can't accept and love her child for who she is, then "there's the door." In their study of families with transgender members, Kuvalanka et al. (2014) reported that even though some extended family members are hesitant or even resistant at first, most eventually become accepting and supportive. Sometimes, grandparents are more supportive than the parents. I had several grandparents participate in our parent support group, either because the parents worked at night and were unable to attend or because they were more supportive than the parents, and they wanted to know how best to be helpful to the family and their transgender or gender expansive grandchild.

2.4 Spouses, Parents, and Children of Transgender Adults

Parents, spouses, and children may go through the stages of grief in coming to terms with those who come out as transgender or gender expansive as adults. Veldorale-Griffin (2014) found that transgender parents and their adult children described their experiences as stressful. The kinds of stress recalled by the children who were adults at the time of this study included bullying at school, having to adjust their view of and ways of talking about their parent, changing pronouns, and feeling pressured to take sides in their parents' conflicts. Stresses reported by the transgender parents included concerns about disclosure to their children, worries about harassment and discrimination at work, and impacts on the family's financial security.

When individuals come out in mid- or late-adulthood, cisgender spouses and/or children (including adult children) are often shaken. Some spouses successfully adapt to the changes associated with their partner's transition and maintain their love and commitments to stay together and manage to make it work; for others, such adjustments and accommodations seem too difficult. Feelings of betrayal and humiliation, sometimes coupled with worries about sexual attraction and intimacy, future financial viability, and effects on the well-being of their children, lead some spouses to pursue divorce (Carlozzi, 2019). If minor children are involved, custody and visitation battles might occur, leaving the transgender or gender expansive spouse vulnerable to discrimination in the courts (Carlozzi, 2017; Stotzer et al., 2014). Such experiences can be agonizing for transgender or gender expansive spouses who love their children and wish to continue to fulfill their parental role and responsibilities. Even when decisions are made to divorce, many divorcing couples maintain a supportive and mutually empathic connection, and they work out custody and visitation agreements that are in the best interests of their children. Some divorcing couples maintain a close friendship and in time come to acknowledge that the person they married is still the same person with whom they share children and/or a relationship history that is important to them.

Similar to younger children tending to be more accepting of a sibling's transition, younger children seem to be more accepting of a parent's transition, while older children and adult children may find acceptance and affirmation more difficult, at least early in their parent's coming out process. Stotzer et al. (2014) suggest that further research is needed to determine parent-child relationship issues that are related to age of the parent when they transition, age of the children when their parent transitions, the children's and the parent's gender, socioeconomic status, fears, and actual incidences of discrimination, and whether the parent is transgender or gender expansive. Stotzer et al. (2014) also reported that studies on children of transgender parents have yielded "no evidence that having a transgender parent affects a child's gender identity or sexual orientation development, nor has an impact on other developmental milestones" (p. 2).

2.5 Intersecting Identities

It is important to acknowledge that the experiences and concerns of transgender and gender expansive persons and their families, as well the treatment options available to them, are often affected or influenced by various intersecting identities, such as age, gender, race/ethnicity, socioeconomic status, religious affiliation/religiosity, and geographic location. A child at Tanner Stage 1 (birth to the start of puberty) may have different concerns than a child or teen at Tanner Stage 2 (onset of puberty) who may seek (with parental support) medical interventions, such as puberty suppressing medications, beyond but including the social supports that the younger child may need (Mahfouda et al., 2017). Teens (with parental permission) or adults who have already gone through puberty might want to pursue gender affirming hormone treatment (GAHT). Ryan et al. (2010) underscored the ways in which race/ethnicity and culture can affect the experiences of LGBT youth, and Singh et al. (2017) suggest that transgender persons of color and transgender persons outside of the United States are more likely than others to experience poverty, health disparities, violence, and less access to health care. Religious affiliation/religiosity is another intersecting identity that can impact the self-acceptance and social treatment of transgender and gender expansive persons. In their study of LGBT young adults, Ryan et al. (2010) found that conservative religious affiliation negatively affected family acceptance, but progressive religious affiliation provided much needed social support for transgender youth and their families. The point is that intersecting identities can affect experiences of transgender and gender expansive persons, the ways in which they are treated, as well as treatment access and options.

In summary, the struggle associated with coming out for transgender or gender expansive persons and their families must not be underestimated. There are emotional hurdles and contextual challenges even for the most supportive and affirming families. There are many tests of the adaptability and resilience of any family system in a family's life cycle, and having a child, spouse, or parent come out as transgender or gender expansive is a formidable test of the family's strength, resilience, and love. The more resilient a family is to begin with, the more equipped they are to metabolize a seeming change in the gender identity of a loved one. Henry et al. (2015) refer to this process as the acting of the *family stress response system* that emerges and orchestrates regulatory processes that balance stability and change in family resilience processes. Affirmative mental health and medical care, as well as support and affirmation by other individuals and support systems, can help bolster the family's resilience.

2.6 Counseling and Support

Those family members who seek support from a mental health professional and/or a support group (which are the people with whom I am most familiar), can get help transitioning from grief, worry, and fear to acceptance and even advocacy for their transgender and gender expansive loved ones. In a study of identity development of transgender youth, Katz-Wize et al. (2017) found that while caregivers are crucial in providing affirming support for their child, "access to additional sources of support can further insulate a child from marginalization and trauma and also provide much-needed support for caregivers themselves" (p.259). Support groups and organizations, such as Parents and Friends of Lesbians and Gays (PFLAG), can provide information and support for family members who are struggling to understand, accept, and affirm their loved one's transition, and also help them realize that they are not alone.

Professional counseling for transgender and gender expansive persons and their families can help parents, spouses, and children make accommodating adjustments to the changes and challenges they are experiencing in their families. Mental health professionals who are affirming and who have appropriate training and/or experience in the provision of care for this population can offer information, cultivate empathy, and promote support for the family member who is transgender or gender expansive, as well as show empathy and support for family members who are experiencing grief or worry. They can help family members get comfortable using the chosen name and pronoun that the transgender or gender expansive person asserts is a proper reflection of their genuine gender self. They can encourage family members to be intentional about using the proper name and pronouns, while also encouraging the transgender or gender expansive person to be patient and recognize that using different names and pronouns takes time to learn, and that even with practice and intentionality, mistakes sometimes happen.

Professional counseling can help the families explore options for coming out and disclosure to others outside of the nuclear family, address school or workplace concerns, and consider how best to respond to incidences of discrimination, harassment, bullying, microaggression, and physical assault. Counseling can be helpful in addressing concerns about co-occurring symptoms, such as depression and anxiety, self-harm, substance abuse, eating disorders, and suicidal ideation and/or attempts. Acceptance or rejection by the family's religious community and sexual experiences and behaviors of the transgender or gender expansive person are sometimes matters about which families want help. Mental health professionals need training in the provision of affirmative care to understand and treat this population competently. The World Professional Association for Transgender

Health (WPATH) provides excellent training opportunities for mental health and medical professionals, and other training opportunities may be available that are offered by WPATH-trained professionals. WPATH Standards of Care, Version 8 (Coleman et al., 2022), is an important resource and guide for competent and ethical treatment of transgender and gender diverse persons.

Mental health professionals can provide referral options for medical care from qualified medical professionals known to be affirming and supportive. They can provide information and/or referrals for facial and body hair removal and for voice training for transgender and gender expansive persons seeking to feminize their voice and appearance, as well as provide information and/or referral regarding the procedures for changing legal documents, such as driver's licenses, passports, and birth certificates. They can also suggest reading materials and online resources to help family members understand what is happening to their loved one and their family and realize that they are not alone. There are many excellent books that can be suggested to family members who are seeking to educate themselves (e.g., Andrews, 2014; Brill & Kenney, 2016; Brill & Pepper, 2008; Carlozzi & Choate, 2019; Hill, 2014).

For parents who have younger children who are engaged in a process of exploring their gender identity, mental health professionals can model openness, calm, and acceptance of the child's exploration, encouraging parents to assume a position of not knowing where the child might land in their exploration (Ehrensaft, 2019), a kind of "benign agnosticism," rather than projecting surplus anxiety into this process of exploration. Considerations regarding medical interventions, such as puberty-suppressing medications, gender-affirming hormone treatments and surgeries can be thoroughly explored and discussed with a qualified mental health professional, and resources for information and provision of such medical interventions can also be discussed.

Mental health professionals may be asked to provide a letter that addresses their assessment of the transgender or gender expansive person's appropriateness and readiness for a medical intervention. Many medical service and health insurance providers require such letters, especially for puberty blockers for transgender youth and for many surgical interventions. Mental health professionals must determine if they meet the qualifying standards and must know what to include in such letters. It is important that qualified mental health professionals receive training in the provision of these assessments and that they follow the guidelines established in the WPATH Standards of Care, Version 8, which can be found on the WPATH website (www.wpath.org).

Just as transgender and gender expansive persons benefit from their participation in support groups, so can family members who participate in a parent or family support group realize that they have some shared experiences with other families. New group participants learn a great deal from parents who are further down the road toward acceptance and advocacy. Parents often serve as resources for support and information for one another (Hillier & Tong, 2019). Knowledgeable and well-trained mental health professionals who may be facilitating a support group can provide accurate information about gender identity, transition, and coming out, and they can assist parents and their children in determining when and how to come out to others in the extended family, school, religious community, and elsewhere. Such support helps family members not only become more accepting, but also builds their strength and resolve to show others that they support their transgender or gender expansive loved one. In the support group for parents that I co-facilitated, it was common for parents to lay bare their concerns and challenges and to share their triumphs in advocating for their transgender or gender expansive child. I have been privileged to witness parents and other family members move from being grief-stricken and frightened to becoming empowered advocates for their child and their family.

2.7 Conclusion

In my private practice, I worked with transgender and gender expansive youth, along with their parents and siblings, and with transgender adults, individually and/or with their spouses and children, helping families transition from fear and sometimes shame, to acceptance and affirmation of their transgender or gender expansive family member, and ultimately move forward in their development as a family to pride and advocacy. I witnessed similar growth in family acceptance, resilience, and advocacy in my work with the parent support group. So, what can we do as mental health professionals? Whether providing counseling or facilitating support groups, we can provide support, education, and information to family members; help them cultivate empathy for one another; help them grow their acceptance, affirmation, and their sense of pride in the adaptability and resilience of their family; and support them in their advocacy efforts on behalf of their transgender child, spouse or parent, or even their ex-spouse if divorced. The pace of this movement from fear and shame to acceptance, affirmation, and advocacy varies, and there are times when the road seems bumpy with steps taken backward and then forward. In their own time, at their own pace, with professional and peer support, most family members come to see this as a movement toward growth, pride, and resilience. In conclusion, my experiences suggest that providing support and affirmative care to transgender and gender expansive persons and their families cultivates greater acceptance, affirmation, resilience, and pride in all, and often leads family members feeling called to serve as advocates for their transgender/gender expansive loved ones. Mental health professionals can become involved in advocacy efforts themselves, as well as suggest avenues for advocacy and activism that families can consider. In addition to becoming active with state organizations that promote laws and policies that support LGBTQ+ civil rights (e.g.,, Oklahomans for Equality and Freedom Oklahoma and similar organizations in other states), they can stay connected to work being done to support the rights and well-being of transgender and gender expansive persons everywhere.

2.8 Organizations of Interest

Below is listed just a few of organizations and their websites at the national and international level that work to advance the rights and wellness of transgender and gender expansive persons:

- World Professional Association for Transgender Health: www.wpath.org
- National Center for Transgender Equality: http://www.transequality.org/
- American Psychological Association and Association for Lesbian, Gay, Bisexual, and Transgender Issues in Counseling Guidelines: https://www.apa.org/practice/guidelines/transgender.pdf
- https://www.counselingsource/competencies/algbtic_competencies.pdf?sfvrsn=8
- Center for Gender Sanity: www.gendersanity.com
- Transgender Law and Policy Institute: http://www.transgenderlaw.org/
- International Foundation for Gender Education: http://www.ifge.org
- Transgender Student Rights at School: http://www.transequality.org/know-your-rights/schools
- Freedom for All Americans: www.fredomforallamericans.org

Questions for Thought and Discussion

1. What concerns are fairly common for parents and other family members of transgender children and teens?
2. Where can family members find support as they struggle to understand, accept, and affirm their transgender and gender expansive loved ones?
3. From what sources can helping professionals learn about best practices for treating transgender persons and their families?
4. In what specific ways can helping professionals be helpful to, and promote resilience in, transgender and gender diverse persons and their families?

Conflict of Interest I have no known conflict of interest to disclose

References

Andrews, A. (2014). *Some assembly required: The not-so-secret life of a transgender teen*. Simon & Schuster.

Brill, S., & Kenney, L. (2016). *The transgender teen: A handbook for parents and professionals supporting transgender and non-binary teens*. Cleis Press.

Brill, S. A., & Pepper, R. (2008). *The transgender child*. Cleis Press.

Bryant, A., & Young, E. (2019). Transgender politics: The civil rights of transgender persons. In A. Carlozzi & K. Choate (Eds.), *Transgender and gender diverse persons: A handbook for service providers, educators, and families* (pp. 71–91). Routledge.

Carlozzi, A. (2017). Counseling transgender persons and their families. *Counseling Today, 60*(2), 44–49.

Carlozzi, A. (2019). Families of transgender and gender diverse persons. In A. Carlozzi & K. Choate (Eds.), *Transgender and gender diverse persons: A handbook for service providers, educators, and families* (pp. 137–158). Routledge.

Carlozzi, A., & Choate, K. (Eds.). (2019). *Transgender and gender diverse persons: A handbook for service providers, educators, and families*. Routledge.

Coleman, E., Radix, A., Bouman, W., Brown, G., de Vries, A., Deutsch, M., Ettner, R., Fraser, L., Goodman, M., Green, J., Hancock, A., Johnson, T., Karasic, D., Knudson, G., Leibowitz, S., Meyer-Bahlburg, H., Monstrey, S., Motmans, J., Nahata, L., et al. (2022). Standards of care for the health of transgender and gender diverse people, version 8. *International Journal of Transgender Health, 23*(S1), S1–S260. https://doi.org/10.1080/26895269.2022.210064

Ehrensaft, D. (2019). Helping transgender and gender diverse youth. In A. Carlozzi & K. Choate (Eds.), *Transgender and gender diverse persons: A handbook for service providers, educators, and families* (pp. 117–136). Routledge.

Grossman, A., D'Augelli, A., & Salter, N. (2011). Male-to-female transgender youth: Gender expression milestones, gender atypicality, victimization, and parents' responses. *Journal of GLBT Family Studies, 2*, 71–92.

Henry, C. S., Morris, A. S., & Harrist, A. W. (2015). Family resilience: Moving into the third wave. *Family Relations, 64*(1), 22–43. https://doi.org/10.1111/fare.12106

Hill, K. (2014). *Rethinking normal: A memoir in transition*. Simon & Schuster.

Hillier, A., & Tong, E. (2019). Parent participation in a support group for families with transgender and gender-nonconforming children: "Being in the company of others who do not question the reality of our experience". *Transgender Health, 4*(10), 168–175. https://doi.org/10.1089/trgh.2018.0018

James, S., Herman, J., Rankin, S., Keisling, M., Mottet, L., & Anafi, M. (2016). *The report of the 2015 U.S. transgender survey*. National Center for Transgender Equality.

Katz-Wise, S., Budge, S., Fugate, E., Flanagan, K., Touloumtzis, C., Rood, B., Perez-Brumer, A., & Leibowitz, S. (2017). Transactional pathways of transgender identity development in transgender and gender nonconforming youth and caregiver perspectives from the trans youth family study. *International Journal of Transgenderism, 18*, 243–263.

Keo-Meier, C., & Ehrensaft, D. (Eds.). (2018). The gender affirmative model: An interdisciplinary approach to supporting transgender and gender expansive children. Washington, D.C.: American Psychological Association.

Kubler-Ross, E. (1970). *On death and dying*. Collier Books/Macmillan.

Kuvalanka, K., Weiner, J., & Mahan, D. (2014). Child, family, and community transformations: Findings from interviews with mothers of transgender girls. *Journal of GLBT Family Studies, 10*, 354–379.

Lev, A., & Alie, L. (2012). Transgender and gender nonconforming children and youth: Developing culturally competent systems of care. In S. Fisher, J. Poirier, & G. Blau (Eds.), *Improving emotional and behavioral outcomes for LGBT youth: A guide for professionals* (pp. 43–66). Brookes.

Mahfouda, S., Moore, J., Siafarikas, A., Zepf, F., & Lin, A. (2017). Puberty suppression in transgender children and adolescents. *The Lancet, 5*, 816–826. https://doi.org/10.1016/S2213-8587(17)30099-2

Ryan, C., Russell, S., Huebner, D., Diaz, R., & Sanchez, J. (2010). Family acceptance in adolescence and health of LGBT young adults. *Journal of Child and Adolescent Psychiatric Nursing, 23*, 205–213.

Singh, A., Hwahng, S., Chang, S., & White, B. (2017). Affirmative counseling with trans/gender variant people of color. In A. Singh & L. Dickey (Eds.), *Affirmative counseling and psychological practice with transgender and gender nonconforming clients* (pp. 41–68). American Psychological Association.

Stotzer, R., Herman, J., & Hasenbush, A. (2014). *Transgender parenting: A review of existing research*. The Williams Institute.

Veldorale-Griffin, A. (2014). Transgender parents and their adult children's experiences of disclosure and transition. *Journal of GLBT Family Studies, 10*, 475–501.

Chapter 3
Building a Family: An Exploration of Queer Resilience Through the Formation of Family

Tangela Roberts, Sarah Haueisen, Aaron D. Jones, Grace Yensch, and Tatyana Smith

3.1 Introduction

SGM (sexual and gender minorities) in rural areas, particularly those with an intersecting minority identity (e.g., a Black racial identity) and/or those identifying as transgender or non-binary gender, have been understudied. They may experience positive relationships within their communities while also experiencing discrimination and oppression from those same communities. This chapter will introduce the concepts of families of origin and families of choice for SGM people in rural areas. Additionally, we will discuss the role of minority stress and highlight the need for a better understanding of rural SGM people. We will then share the results of a related qualitative study of rural SGM students and the implications of the research findings.

3.2 Families of Origin

A family of origin typically consists of one's parents, siblings, partners, children, grandparents, and extended biological or adoptive family. Families of origin can be a source of both support and distress; therefore, it is essential to understand how family dynamics influence the lives of sexual and gender minorities (SGM), especially SGM youth.

Research has consistently shown that having supportive parents and families can have positive health outcomes for SGM youth. SGM youth with supportive families

T. Roberts (✉) · S. Haueisen · A. D. Jones · G. Yensch · T. Smith
Department of Counselor Education and Counseling Psychology, Western Michigan University, Kalamazoo, MI, USA
e-mail: tangela.roberts@wmich.edu

J. M. Koch et al. (eds.), *Identity as Resilience in Minoritized Communities*, Emerging Issues in Family and Individual Resilience,
https://doi.org/10.1007/978-3-031-38977-1_3

are less likely to experience depression, anxiety, and suicidal ideation compared to those without supportive families (Eisenberg & Resnick, 2006; Ryan et al., 2009, 2010). Supportive families are also related to increased health-promoting behaviors for SGM youth, such as exercising regularly and eating a healthy diet (Eisenberg & Resnick, 2006). In general, SGM youth with supportive families are more likely to have positive self-esteem and to feel good about themselves (Ryan et al., 2010).

Unsupportive family of origin environments may have detrimental effects on the health of sexual minorities. Lack of family support may be a significant factor in substance abuse and psychological distress, including feelings of rejection from family and peers (McGeough & Sterzing, 2018). Parental and familial support of SGM youth has been associated with lower reported daily negative affect (Kiekens & Mereish, 2022), worry, anxiety, depression, and substance use concerns (Hubachek et al., 2023; Milton & Knutson, 2021; Ryan et al., 2010).

Evidence suggests a family systems approach may be an effective framework of treatment when working with sexual minorities, further emphasizing the role of the family of origin and choice in the well-being of sexual minority youth (Jacobs & Freundlich, 2006; McGeough & Sterzing, 2018). The family systems approach focuses on the general function of the family unit rather than individuals and their roles within the family, prioritizing awareness of problems in overall family functioning over individual behaviors. Understanding family systems in which SGM youth are situated may help us better understand the experiences of SGM youth (Jacobs & Freundlich, 2006; McGeough & Sterzing, 2018). Acknowledgment of unsupportive behaviors in the family that may result in negative health consequences for SGM youth allows the opportunity for modification.

3.3 Families of Choice

Chosen families, or nonbiological kinship bonds, may be an essential source of social support for SGM individuals. While chosen families may also have similar characteristics to families of origin in structure and members' roles, research has revealed that family structures may hold differential meanings for individuals of diverse sexual orientations or gender identities; specifically, SGM people have found their family of origin's opinions on their relationships less critical than they did friends' opinions (Blair & Pukall, 2015; Muraco, 2006). Research has also been conducted on how individuals create and conceptualize their chosen families. For the formation and maintenance of chosen families, Oswald (2002) found that intentionality in family creation and redefinition of the family were essential processes for gay and lesbian members of chosen families. While chosen families may also have similar characteristics to families of origin in terms of structure and roles of members, a study of gay and lesbian individuals involved in chosen families revealed that there might be variance in the perceived meaning of family structures based on sexual orientation and gender identity (Muraco, 2006). Many SGM people endorse participation in a chosen family; however, few report chosen family as their only family and often include the family of origin in their definitions of a family (Hull & Ortyl, 2019). Soler et al. (2018) explored the nature of families of choice of young adult gay and bisexual cisgender men. While the majority (63%) of participants reported having chosen a family, 88% included a family of origin in their definition of family. However, SGM members of chosen families may attribute their participation in a chosen family to insufficiency in their families of origin (Braithwaite et al., 2010). SGM tend to rely more on peer support than on support from their family of origin, often viewing friends' opinions as more crucial than family (Dewaele et al., 2011; Blair & Pukall, 2015).

Participation in a chosen family may affect an individual's well-being, often protecting them from the negative ramifications of discrimination (Hailey et al., 2020; Haines et al., 2018). Inclusion in chosen families was a protective factor against psychological distress for Black SGM youth, promoting resilience and belongingness (Hailey et al., 2020; Levitt et al., 2015). Drabble et al. (2018) found that SGM women identified peer support and chosen family as essential aspects of coping and resilience. There is a lack of research focusing exclusively on the experiences of transgender people in chosen families. Still, Muzzey et al. (2021) found that transmasculine and nonbinary youth reported their chosen family as an essential source of support during their chosen name transition. Further research should be conducted to understand the specific nature of chosen families for transgender individuals.

3.4 Minority Stress

Experiences of support for SGM youth are compounded by the number of minority stressors they experience, which is increasingly important for SGM with racially diverse identities and/or those in resource-poor areas (i.e., low-income, rural, or politically hostile areas). Minority stressors result from social oppression stress, above and beyond the everyday stress experienced by the general population, further increasing health disparities among minority populations (Brooks, 1981). When SGM people do not conform to heteronormative expectations – such as that they should identify as heterosexual, enter relationships with people of the "opposite" gender, and conform to gender norms (Drabble, 2018; Hailey et al., 2020; Masten, 2007) – they face discrimination, victimization, and other forms of violence. More specifically, experiences of homophobia and external stressors related to one's sexuality may lead to increased internalized homophobia, prejudice against sexual minorities, and decreased ability to find healthy coping mechanisms in one's community. These minority stressors may lead to increased psychological distress, such as depression and anxiety, and increased suicidal ideations or attempts compared to their heterosexual counterparts (Fish et al., 2020; Hailey et al., 2020). Educators and mental health professionals need to consider the impact of minority stressors, such as internalized homophobia, on the health and well-being of SGM students (Brooks, 1981; Fish et al., 2020; Hailey et al., 2020).

3.5 Coming Out

For many SGM youth, one of the first hurdles to living one's truth comes in sexual orientation disclosure (i.e., coming out to self and others). Coming out is a developmental process. This means that the coming out process does not end when the individual starts expressing their sexuality to others. With every new encounter, new environment, or new person, SGM people constantly disclose their identity (i.e., constantly coming out) to others (D'Augelli et al., 2010; Kiekens & Mereish 2022; Muzzey et al., 2021). Family, in both a traditional sense (i.e., biological family) and chosen family (i.e., close friends, loved ones, and other supporters), plays a significant role in the experiences of coming out and resilience among SGM youth.

3.5.1 Coming Out to Family of Origin

For most SGM youth, there is a two-year difference between when an SGM youth self-identifies with a minority sexual or gender identity (i.e., coming out to self) and when their parents become aware of their child's SGM identity or coming out to others (D'Augelli et al., 2010). This indicates many SGM youth are engaging in years-long identity concealment, which is related to increased anxiety, depression, risky sexual behaviors, and isolation (D'Augelli et al., 2010; Dewaele et al., 2011). SGM youth further in their sexual orientation development tend to have a better psychosocial adjustment (D'Augelli et al., 2010). Those who experience support from their family (of origin or choice) have better outcomes when coming out to their families of origin (D'Augelli et al., 2010; Dewaele et al., 2011; Levitt et al., 2015).

3.5.2 Coming Out in Rural America

SGM youth in different regional contexts may experience and report outness differently. Rural culture in the United States is often associated with conservative religious and political values, an affinity for solid kinship ties, elevated levels of visibility, and an emphasis on challenging work and self-sufficiency; still, rural culture is neither static nor homogeneous (Glon et al., 2021; Oswald & Culton, 2003; Roberts et al., 2022). Although SGM in rural areas report thriving affirmative friendships and family relationships, community tolerance often disguises anti-LGBTQ+ sentiments, lack of equal rights, and hostile attitudes (Oswald & Culton, 2003). Rural schools are often less receptive to implementing SGM-specific programming, leaving SGM students in rural areas without the opportunity to obtain support and develop communities that may become their families of choice (Roberts et al., 2022). However, social media has mitigated some deficiencies to increase access to individuals in rural areas (Glon et al., 2021; Li et al., 2015; Oswald & Culton, 2003; Owens et al., 2023). Geographic isolation, an insufficient opportunity to socialize with other SGM, and the perceived need to conceal gender or sexual identities can contribute to mental distress, lack of social support, and fewer visible SGM role models in rural areas.

3.6 Method

This chapter presents a thematic analysis of interviews with four SGM students. Within our analysis of the interviews, we explore the concept of family and resilience with SGM youth. We conducted interviews in 2020 as part of a research study that explored aspects of minority stress within the phenomenon of identifying as an SGM in a rural high school (Roberts et al., 2022). In this chapter, we focus specifically on the concepts of family of origin, family of choice, and resilience related to the perceived experiences of SGM youth. We purposefully selected participants who shared a homogeneous experience of a particular condition, event, or situation. Therefore, all participants in the current study identified as SGM were currently enrolled as a college or graduate student, and were raised in a rural Midwestern area. Data were collected in February 2020 at a regional event for SGM students, and all participants provided informed consent for their participation. This study was approved by the first author's Institutional Review Board.

3.6.1 The Research Team

The analytic team for this study consisted of one psychologist and three counseling psychology graduate students interested in race and other issues of diversity within psychology. The primary investigators were one psychologist (an African American bisexual cisgender woman) and one educator (an African American heterosexual cisgender woman). As a research team, we met to discuss our reflexive thoughts and feelings about GSM in rural areas. As a group, we identified our perceptions of rural areas as hostile to SGM communities (especially for SGM communities of color), a perception of rural areas as resource-poor, and a general equation of rural with White.

3.6.2 Participants

We recruited four SGM students at a regional event for SGM students. Names were changed to pseudonyms to protect participant confidentiality. One participant identified as African American and three identified as White. All but one participant named their gender as non-binary. They ranged in age from 22 to 29 and were current undergraduate or graduate students at various Midwestern colleges and universities. The four people interviewed included: Terrance – a 29-year-old, Black, queer-identified, non-binary transmasculine agnostic person; Nick – a 24-year-old, White, gay-identified, cisgender man who identifies as a non-denominational Christian theist; Reeves – a 28-year-old, White, bisexual-identified, assigned female at birth (AFAB) trans man who is non religious; and Finley – a 22-year-old, White, queer-identified, non-binary, assigned female at birth (AFAB) femme who identifies as pagan/spiritual.

3.6.3 *Procedures*

The data presented within this chapter are part of a more extensive study in which we examined minority stress experiences for rural SGM students. We analyzed interview data to explore family experiences (i.e., a family of origin and family of choice) and resilience as described by SGM students. A semi-structured interview included open-ended and non-leading questions. While not required, all participants previously attended K-12 education in rural areas. Having attended rural schools may have influenced participants' perspectives because they may have been more comfortable sharing their experiences in an SGM-affirmative environment. To be included in the study, participants had to be over 18, self-identify as SGM, and be currently enrolled as undergraduate or graduate students. Four SGM students were interviewed, and their responses are detailed in this chapter.

The first two authors conducted interviews via Zoom. All participants engaged in one interview with the primary investigators and agreed to be contacted if further information was needed. Interviews ranged from 58 to 101 min (M = 79 min). Interviews were audio-recorded and transcribed verbatim. Researchers used memo writing during and after the interviews to further acknowledge researcher reflexivity. In analyzing student interviews, we took a descriptive approach to inquiry and allowed coding categories to appear from the analysis (Willig, 2014). In doing so, we explored the phenomenon of family (i.e., family of origin and family of choice) and resiliency experienced by SGM students. All data have been anonymized to protect participant confidentiality.

3.7 Results

The following section will discuss the results of interviews with the four SGM students. These results are divided into four main sections: the family of origin experiences, the family of choice experiences, living as SGM in rural areas, and resilience experiences.

3.7.1 Family of Origin Experiences

Family of origin typically consists of parents, siblings, partners, children, grandparents, and extended biological or adoptive family. Consistent with this conceptualization, the SGM students we interviewed described interactions with siblings, partners, parents, children, and extended family. Participants described positive and negative experiences within their families of origin. An example of positive experiences with families was SGM students felt their family strongly desired to keep them safe in a world rampant with heterosexism and violence. Examples of negative experiences included SGM students dealing with family members' heterosexism and lack of an affirmative environment. Below are excerpts and explanations of participants' responses related to this topic:

> I think my mom has always been the biggest person I want to impress the most...after (coming out to mom), I honestly didn't care what anyone else thought. Addressing that with the most important person to me at that moment was the journey. The journey was to disclose to my mother, not necessarily come out two everyone else. That was my identity once that conversation happened. – *Terrance, 29 y/o Black queer non-binary transman.*

> I had distinct memories of sitting on my porch in the middle of summer with my aunt and mom for hours, talking about queerness. They were so curious and just wanted to know more so they could do better. I learned (queer history) talking to them about it and just learned it from conversing with them. Once I had a level of like comfortability with them... I went full force, full force gay. – *Finley, 22 y/o White queer, non-binary femme.*

> [Mom] was afraid that if anyone learned I was gay, some violence could target me, so I had that fear from her flowing into me. My reaction to that was not to say anything. I felt unsafe; I felt I was guarding this secret that something terrible could transpire against me. – *Nick, 24 y/o White gay cisgender man.*

Participants expressed positive and negative perceptions and experiences within their families of origin. Regarding their positive experiences, our participants described the joy of teaching their parents and children about SGM culture and history; support from the family of origin after coming out; using family to curate an SGM-affirmative space for themselves and others; feeling a sense of strength after receiving positive responses from mothers to coming out; and connecting with and seeking strength from other SGM family members. Participants reported the following negative experiences: receiving heterosexist messages from school; receiving insufficient support from the family of origin; and experiencing fear of coming out to the family. Participants mentioned being aware of their parents' fears about their child coming out in a heterosexist society, which related to their decision not to come out to others.

3.7.2 Family of Choice Experiences

Family of choice has been described as close connections with non-relatives, such as fictive kinship networks, friends, classmates, colleagues, and community members. The participants all identified that their current family of choice consisted of classmates, friends, members of student organizations (e.g., Gender & Sexualities Alliance [GSA], social justice student clubs, or feminist student clubs), and SGM affirmative teachers and school staff. The participants also discussed finding a family of choice while attending college in cities perceived as more SGM affirmative than their small rural hometowns. Avenues to obtain access to this future family of choice included searching for SGM affirmative colleges, joining (or starting) SGM organizations at their intended colleges, and finding jobs located within queer community spaces (e.g., café, drag show, community center, social services). Below are excerpts and explanations of participants' responses related to this theme.

> There wasn't an official LGBT (lesbian, gay, bisexual, transgender)-anything at my high school until I was about to leave, but a group of LGBT kids and allies would informally hang out. Even though I hadn't come out, even to them, I would hang out with them. It was a good experience to be in that atmosphere and see that, as you know, maybe I could exist as someone. And many of my fears and worries didn't have to control my life. I guess. – *Nick, 24 y/o White gay cisgender man.*

> It's hard to even in (nearby mid-sized city) because I work with many trans people. I don't want to invade their spaces, be unable to disclose my stuff, and then have them worry. (I ask myself) should I disclose all this stuff in front of you? Technically, I don't think I have a community, but my husband's also trans, and he's bisexual or pansexual. So it does make it a little bit easier to come home and talk to them about a lot of the stuff that I'm going through, which is nice. – *Reeves, 28 y/o White bisexual non-binary trans man.*

> I'm learning about asking for help, and I'm learning about trusting that other people want to be involved in my life and collaborate and do what's best for me or, you know, to help me achieve a certain goal. I'm learning to trust that it's not always from a blood family. The notion of chosen family, particularly within a queer context, has been heavy on my mind and has aided my healing. – *Terrance, 29 y/o Black queer, non-binary transmasculine person.*

Within the theme of the family of choice, participants generally reported positive experiences. They described using their school's gay-straight alliance (GSA) group to work through internalized heterosexism, gain strength and validation from other queer students, seek queer family at work or in college, discover advocates among schoolteachers and staff, find inspiration from visibly queer students, and generally be immersed in SGM culture as a form of healing, strength, and resiliency. Although many family of choice connections developed within a school context (high school or college), several of our participants wanted to keep those connections even after school ended. Negative experiences reported within the theme of the family of choice included a lack of queer role models. Participants also noted a shared perception of college as a safe environment to explore one's sexual orientation and gender identity and make strategic plans to come out in college.

3.7.3 *Living as an SGM Youth in a Rural Area*

All participants indicated a desire, to some extent, to leave their rural areas for suburban or urban areas that were outwardly perceived to be more SGM affirmative (e.g., Chicago, Los Angeles, New York, Toronto). Below are excerpts and explanations of participants' responses related to their life within a rural context.

> It was a predominantly White school in a predominantly White town. The kind of town with two major high schools. And then, both housing projects fed into my school and the city's richest middle school. You know, this is where you're going to school with people whose families owned the town like there are three main names everyone knows. – *Terrance, 29 y/o Black queer, non-binary transmasculine person.*

> The way I was socialized, I come from a smaller rural town, what I was feeling at the time was that it's like if anyone finds out about that or it came out, it seemed like to me it would have been the end of the world, so that was the mindset I was living in…Once I just got out of that cage of worry, I wasn't sure how to even begin to (date) or anything like that…because everything that has been taught about was so tailored through a more heteronormative perspective. – *Nick, 24 y/o White Cisgender gay man.*

> I love the town's schools, and I think they did a really good job with what they were given. Definitely better than friends who went to (a neighboring town). So, they definitely did a better job than many other places, but it still was harmful. – *Finley, 22 y/o White queer, non-binary femme.*

Our participants seemed conflicted about living in rural areas, which they described as small insular communities. On the one hand, they recognized (and identified) instances of antagonism toward minority sexual orientations and gender identities, as well as a fear of being outed; on the other hand, they seemed to reject the notion of having to go outside the home environment to obtain support. As one participant said, "I feel like I'm stuck in this small rural town, but I'm not moving because my family anchors me here" – *Reeves, 28 y/o White bisexual non-binary trans man.*

3.7.4 *Advocacy and Resilience Experiences*

Resilience refers to an individual's ability to adapt and cope in the face of adversity, such as discrimination, trauma, or stress (Masten, 2007). It involves developing skills and resources that allow individuals to overcome challenges and maintain a sense of well-being. For LGBTQ youth, resilience can involve building a positive sense of self, developing a supportive social network, and accessing resources to address discrimination and other challenges that may arise (Drabble et al., 2018; Levitt et al., 2015; Oswald, 2002). The following quotes relate to participants' experiences of resilience.

> I brought acceptance to myself because I strongly advocated for other queer people before I came out to myself. I thought I was a great ally, but truth be told, I was just gay. I learned a lot about this stuff and was like studying it – *Finley, 22 y/o White queer, non-binary femme.*

> I think it's a lot of understanding my own worth and understanding that it's going to be a hard road, but ultimately is it worth that? And yes, obviously, it's worth it! Otherwise, I wouldn't be here right now. It's a lot of evaluating the pros and cons, and I would say a lot of it had to do with my upbringing and what constitutes being a female. And like a lot of my hesitation with my transition, I think it mainly was how I didn't want to lose my feminist point of view. And being seen as a White man gives me a lot more privilege, and it kind of sucks because sitting there advocating it, I think it looks different, and it was a struggle of whether I want to give up this portion of me? – *Reeves, 28 y/o White bisexual non-binary trans man.*

Brooks' (1981) theory of minority stress stated that holding minority identities can be associated with positive effects, as seen in the participants' engagement in advocacy. Every participant mentioned outness as a critical way to offer visibility, safety, validation, and support to other SGM people, especially those not out, by modeling an authentic, joyous existence. Participants also described how asserting an identity affiliation could open educational and humanizing personal conversations with others as well as opportunities to stand up for SGM people and issues. Another critical part of advocacy work involved finding resources, becoming involved in communities, and inviting other SGM individuals along as a means of giving back and helping them cope – many times because the participants themselves had not been aware of or had access to these resources and communities earlier in their lives. Other forms of advocacy included creating SGM-related groups, participating in conferences and workshops, and dialoguing about and engaging in intersectional work with other SGM people as a community. In short, taking part in advocacy delivered positive effects such as increased social support, a sense of community, coping skills, strength, and resilience, which are supporting elements of Brooks' (1981) theory of minority stress.

3.8 Discussion

SGM participants in our study were engaged in creating an affirmative family space within their families of origin and their families of choice. While engaging within these spaces, the SGM youth, particularly those in resource-poor areas, were discovering queer families through acts of resilience. While the researchers' previously held assumptions may cast rural areas as places devoid of SGM support, our participants reported a perception of support from the family of origin and family of choice. Participants reported heterosexist experiences within families of origin; however, participants also found value in educating families of origin about SGM identity. Furthermore, some participants found encouragement from families of origin as a catalyst to living more openly. Feedback from participants also demonstrated the formal and informal avenues SGM youth in rural areas take to forming families of choice (e.g., establishing a GSA or seeking out other SGM students in college). When participants perceived a lack of a structured SGM community, they formed meaningful connections with other SGM youth and allies in their peer group.

This chapter provides valuable insight into the experiences of SGM youth that may have implications for healthcare. Clinicians can consider sources of support in their conceptualization of SGM client issues. Mental health clinicians may consider a family of origin and family of choice experiences in working with SGM youth. SGM youth may build a family of choice through connection to other SGM individuals. SGM youth who express a lack of connection with other SGM individuals may benefit from the encouragement of connection to others, such as by providing psychoeducation regarding in-person or online support groups. Aspects of family of origin experience may also be a source of support important for clinicians to assess. For example, SGM youth may experience feelings of agency by teaching their family of origin about SGM identities. Additionally, given the positive experiences expressed by SGM youth engaged in advocacy, clinicians may consider encouraging engagement in advocacy as a strategy for bolstering resilience.

In addition to guidance around support for SGM youth, the study also has implications for individuals working in higher education. Colleges and universities can play an important role in supporting SGM students by providing resources such as campus organizations and other SGM student services. Highlighting these resources allows higher education institutions to create affirmative environments for SGM youth and help them feel hopeful about their future. Finally, the chapter underscores the importance of engagement in policy advocacy at the local, state, and national levels. SGM individuals face unique discrimination, and policies that support SGM people can make a significant difference in their lives. Advocating for policies that support SGM individuals, individuals, and organizations can help create more inclusive communities and support systems.

Although the study provides valuable information on the experiences of SGM youth in rural areas, some limitations should be noted. While the study included one participant who identified as a person of color, additional research is necessary to gain a deeper understanding of the experiences of SGM youth of color. Considering the potentially compounded marginalization that may result from intersecting heterosexism, cissexism, and racism, it is probable that SGM youth of color face distinct challenges and require tailored support. Although this topic was not within the scope of the current study, it is crucial to conduct further research to address the unique needs of this population.

3.9 Conclusion

SGM participants in our study were shaping their homes and families into the image of who and what they need. Throughout this process of actively shaping their family spaces, assistance from mental health providers and supportive community members needs not to focus on ways SGM youth can leave their homes. Instead, we should focus on how they can actively gain support to create the change needed to obtain families that they deserve, need, and want. Relocating to a larger city area or an area known to be openly SGM affirmative is not the answer to the question of how to find a family as an SGM youth. Below, we offer some additional media resources.

3.9.1 *Media Representations of SGM Youth and Families*

- **TV Shows**
  - *Pose* (2018–2021)
    - The series shows the formation of a family of choice and highlights the complexities of coming out to a family of origin by depicting LGBTQ+ people of color in New York City during the 1980s–1990s.
  - *Noah's Arc* (2005–2006)
    - This series shows the detailed lives of four Black gay men in Los Angeles. Throughout the series, we see the formation of a strong family of choice between the four main characters.
  - *I am Jazz* (2015–ongoing)
    - This series highlights the lived experience of a transwoman from adolescence to young adulthood. Within the series, we see a highlight of the importance of having a supportive family of origin throughout the identity development process.
- **Movies**
  - *Pariah* (2011)
    - This movie shows the impact of coming out (or being outed) on one Black lesbian teenager in Brooklyn, NY. The movie shows conflictual relationships with family or origin and a search for an affirmative space.
  - *If These Walls Could Talk 2* (2000)
    - This movie depicts lesbian life in a series of three separate stories. The characters in this movie deal with issues with their family of origin (both in young and older adulthood), positive and negative aspects of a family of choice, and the development of a future family for SGM couples.
  - *Ma Vie en Rose* (1997)
    - This Belgian movie shows a transgender girl and the process of her family of origin accepting her gender identity. The movie shows a family struggling to come to terms with their child's gender identity and the mental health impacts of an unsupportive family.

Questions for Thought and Discussion

1. How might you work with a family who accepts their child's SGM identity but pressures the child to remain closeted because of fears of experiencing harm in a heterosexist world?

2. What resources would you provide for an SGM youth in your area seeking social support? Local resources? National resources? Virtual/online resources?
3. What are some additional ways to foster resilience in rural SGM youth?

Conflict of Interest We have no known conflict of interest to disclose

References

Blair, K. L., & Pukall, C. F. (2015). Family matters, but sometimes chosen family matters more: Perceived social network influence in the dating decisions of same- and mixed-sex couples. *Canadian Journal of Human Sexuality, 24*(3), 257–270. https://doi.org/10.3138/cjhs.243-A3

Braithwaite, D. O., Bach, B. W., Baxter, L. A., DiVerniero, R., Hammonds, J. R., Hosek, A. M., & Wolf, B. M. (2010). Constructing family: A typology of voluntary kin. *Journal of Social and Personal Relationships, 27*(3), 388–407. https://doi.org/10.1177/0265407510361615

Brooks, V. R. (1981). Minority Stress and Lesbian Women. Lexington, MA: Lexington Books.

D'Augelli, A. R., Grossman, A. H., Starks, M. T., & Sinclair, K. O. (2010). Factors associated with parents' knowledge of gay, lesbian, and bisexual youths' sexual orientation. *Journal of GLBT Family Studies, 6*(2), 178–198. https://doi.org/10.1080/15504281003705410

Dewaele, A., Cox, N., Van den Berghe, W., & Vincke, J. (2011). Families of choice? Exploring the supportive networks of lesbians, gay men, and bisexuals. *Journal of Applied Social Psychology, 41*, 312–331. https://doi.org/10.1111/j.1559-1816.2010.00715.x

Drabble, L. A., Trocki, K. F., Salcedo, B., Morales, B. R., & Korcha, R. A. (2018). Strengths and coping strategies in the life narratives of sexual minority women. *Journal of Gay & Lesbian Social Services, 30*(4), 409–429. https://doi.org/10.1080/10538720.2018.1509757

Eisenberg, M. E., & Resnick, M. D. (2006). Suicidality among gay, lesbian and bisexual youth: The role of protective factors. *Journal of Adolescent Health, 39*(5), 662–668. https://doi.org/10.1016/j.jadohealth.2006.04.024

Fish, J. N., McInroy, L. B., Paceley, M. S., Williams, N. D., Henderson, S., Levine, D. S., & Edsall, R. N. (2020). "I'm kinda stuck at home with unsupportive parents right now": LGBTQ youths' experiences with COVID-19 and the importance of online support. *Journal of Adolescent Health, 67*(3), 450–452. https://doi.org/10.1016/j.jadohealth.2020.06.002

Glon, B., Giano, Z., Hubach, R., & Hammer, T. (2021). Rurality, gay-related rejection sensitivity, and mental health outcomes for gay and bisexual men. *Journal of Gay & Lesbian Mental Health, 25*(4), 408–426. https://doi.org/10.1080/19359705.2020.1850595

Hailey, J., Burton, W., & Arscott, J. (2020). We are family: Chosen and created families as a protective factor against racialized trauma and anti-LGBTQ oppression among African American sexual and gender minority youth. *Journal of GLBT Family Studies, 16*(2), 176–191. https://doi.org/10.1080/1550428X.2020.172413

Haines, K. M., Boyer, C. R., Giovanazzi, C., & Galupo, M. P. (2018). "Not a real family": Microaggressions directed toward LGBTQ families. *Journal of Homosexuality, 65*(9), 1138–1151. https://doi.org/10.1080/00918369.2017.1406217

Hubachek, S. Q., Clark, K. A., Pachankis, J. E., & Dougherty, L. R. (2023). Explicit and implicit bias among parents of sexual and gender minority youth. *Journal of Family Psychology, 37*(2), 203–214. https://doi.org/10.1037/fam0001037

Hull, K. E., & Ortyl, T. A. (2019). Conventional and cutting-edge: Definitions of family in LGBT communities. *Sexuality Research & Social Policy: A Journal of the NSRC, 16*(1), 31–43. https://doi.org/10.1007/s13178-018-0324-2

Jacobs, J., & Freundlich, M. (2006). Achieving permanency for LGBTQ youth. Child Welfare, 299–316.

Kiekens, W. J., & Mereish, E. H. (2022). The association between daily concealment and affect among sexual and gender minority adolescents: The moderating role of family and peer support. *Journal of Adolescent Health, 70*(4), 650–657. https://doi.org/10.1016/j.jadohealth.2021.11.019

Levitt, H. M., Horne, S. G., Puckett, J., Sweeney, K. K., & Hampton, M. L. (2015). Gay families: Challenging racial and sexual/gender minority stressors through social support. *Journal of GLBT Family Studies, 11*(2), 173–202. https://doi.org/10.1080/1550428X.2014.958266

Li, M. J., Hubach, R. D., & Dodge, B. (2015). Social milieu and mediators of loneliness among gay and bisexual men in rural Indiana. *Journal of Gay & Lesbian Mental Health, 19*(4), 331–346. https://doi.org/10.1080/19359705.2015.1033798

Masten, A. S. (2007). Resilience in developing systems: Progress and promise as the fourth wave rises. *Development and Psychopathology, 19*(3), 921–930. https://doi.org/10.1017/S0954579407000442

McGeough, B. L. & Sterzing, P. R. (2018). A systematic review of family victimization experiences among Sexual Minority Youth. *The Journal of Primary Prevention, 39*(5), 491–528. https://doi.org/10.1007/s10935-018-0523-x

Milton, D. C., & Knutson, D. (2021). Family of origin, not chosen family, predicts psychological health in an LGBTQ+ sample. *Psychology of Sexual Orientation and Gender Diversity.* Advanced online publication. https://doi.org/10.1037/sgd0000531.

Muraco, A. (2006). Intentional families: Fictive kin ties between cross-gender, different sexual orientation friends. *Journal of Marriage and Family, 68*(5), 1313–1325. https://doi.org/10.1111/j.1741-3737.2006.00330.x

Muzzey, F. K., Kinney, M. K., Maas, M. K., & McCauley, H. L. (2021). Support networks of transmasculine and nonbinary young adults during chosen name transition. *Psychology & Sexuality, 13*(3), 652–662. https://doi.org/10.1016/j.jadohealth.2018.10.227

Oswald, R. F. (2002). Resilience within the family networks of lesbians and gay men: Intentionality and redefinition. *Journal of Marriage and Family, 64*(2), 374–383. https://doi.org/10.1111/j.1741-3737.2002.00374.x

Oswald, R. F., & Culton, L. S. (2003). Under the Rainbow: Rural Gay Life and Its Relevance for Family Providers. *Family Relations, 52*, 72–81. https://doi-org.libproxy.library.wmich.edu/10.1111/j.1741-3729.2003.00072.x

Owens, C., Shrodes, A., Kraus, A., Birnholtz, J., Moskowitz, D. A., & Macapagal, K. (2023). Motivations to start and stop using sexual networking applications among adolescent sexual minority men. *Sexuality Research and Social Policy, 20*, 329–339. https://doi.org/10.1007/s13178-021-00641-3

Roberts, T., Roberts, L., Carpenter, Z., Haueisen, S., Jones, A., Schutte, K., & Smith, T. (2022). Existing in the void: An interpretative phenomenological analysis of rural LGBTQ+ students. *Journal of LGBT Youth*, 1–29. Advance online publication. https://doi.org/10.1080/19361653.2022.2104774.

Ryan, C., Huebner, D., Diaz, R. M., & Sanchez, J. (2009). Family rejection as a predictor of negative health outcomes in white and Latino lesbian, gay, and bisexual young adults. *Pediatrics, 123*(1), 346–352. https://doi.org/10.1542/peds.2007-3524

Ryan, C., Russell, S. T., Huebner, D., Diaz, R., & Sanchez, J. (2010). Family acceptance in adolescence and the health of LGBT young adults. *Journal of Child and Adolescent Psychiatric Nursing, 23*(4), 205–213. https://doi.org/10.1111/j.1744-6171.2010.00246.x

Soler, J. H., Caldwell, C. H., Córdova, D., Harper, G., & Bauermeister, J. A. (2018). Who counts as family? Family typologies, family support, and family undermining among young adult gay and bisexual men. *Sexuality Research & Social Policy: A Journal of the NSRC, 15*(2), 123–138. https://doi.org/10.1007/s13178-017-0288-7

Willig, C. (2014). *Introducing qualitative research in psychology* (2nd ed.). Open University Press.

Chapter 4
Latinx LGBTQ People and Their Families: The Role of Latinx Cultural Values, Beliefs, and Traditions

Roberto L. Abreu, Julio A. Martin, and Koree S. Badio

Latinx LGBTQ people face unprecedented physical and emotional health disparities compared to their White, non-Latinx counterparts (e.g., HIV, substance abuse, mental health disorders) as a result of intersecting oppressive experiences such as racism, xenophobia, cissexism, and heterosexism (e.g., Bostwick et al., 2014; Kann et al., 2018; Ocasio et al., 2016). The COVID-19 pandemic has exacerbated and created new challenges for Latinx people and their families, leading to decreased access to mental health services and increased mental health concerns (Abreu et al., 2023a; Cortés-García et al., 2022; D′ Costa et al., 2021; Harkness et al., 2020; Penner et al., 2021). Moreover, as a result of quarantine and social distancing measures during the COVID-19 pandemic, Latinx families have had to learn new roles in order to support their Latinx LGBTQ loved ones (e.g., providing LGBTQ-specific support), exacerbating potential ruptures within the family unit due to disagreements and misunderstanding about sexuality and gender identity (Abreu et al., 2023a). Taking on such roles is incredibly taxing for Latinx parents and family members who are already facing multiple stressors such as financial and language barriers (Manzano-Sanchez et al., 2019; Victor et al., 2020).

Studies have uncovered the importance of family support in the well-being of LGBTQ people (e.g., Abreu et al., 2022; Needham & Austin, 2010; Ryan et al., 2010; Saewyc et al., 2009). Specific to Latinx LGBTQ people and their families, researchers have observed the importance of specific Latinx cultural values, beliefs, and traditions when working with this community. Specifically, cultural values, beliefs, and traditions directly influence the relationship among Latinx LGBTQ people and their families. Unfortunately, the literature has been slow to provide culturally appropriate clinical implications for working with Latinx parents and

---

R. L. Abreu (✉) · J. A. Martin · K. S. Badio
University of Florida, Gainesville, FL, USA
e-mail: rabreu26@ufl.edu

J. M. Koch et al. (eds.), *Identity as Resilience in Minoritized Communities*, Emerging Issues in Family and Individual Resilience,
https://doi.org/10.1007/978-3-031-38977-1_4

families and their LGBTQ family members. To address these gaps in the literature, using an intersectional approach to understand the experiences of Latinx LGBTQ people and their families, in this chapter we aim to: (a) provide a discussion about different Latinx cultural values, beliefs, and traditions and theoretical frameworks that might be useful in understanding the intersectional experiences of Latinx LGBTQ people and their families, (b) provide a review of the available research about the experiences of Latinx LGBTQ people and their families, and (c) provide recommendations for clinicians working with Latinx LGBTQ people and their families.

4.1 Latinx Cultural Values, Beliefs, and Traditions

Latinx cultural values, beliefs, and traditions are of utmost importance when understanding how Latinx families operate within systems. From a systems view, through the cultural value of *familismo*, or the need to put family members and the collective's needs above that of the individual (Arredondo et al., 2014; Marin & Marin, 1991), one can visualize how for Latinx families caring for one another is of vast importance. For instance, *familismo* guides the understanding that parents need to make decisions that they believe most benefit their child and go to any length to protect their child. *Familismo* helps us know that at the core of parent behavior, there is a desire to do what is best for their child given their understanding of the world, their context, and information that is available to them. Through this lens, one understands that there are cultural strengths to take into consideration when working with Latinx LGBTQ people and their families that are useful in moving family members towards accepting their LGBTQ members.

Gender norms such as *machismo,* or the belief that men within the family unit must present as hypermasculine, removed from emotions, and reject feminine behaviors, and *marianismo,* the belief that Latina women must self-sacrifice for the family's well-being (Gil & Vazquez, 1996; Mayo, 1997; Saez et al., 2010), are both important cultural norms that play out in family relations. From a systems perspective, a Latinx family has specific roles within their subsystems that are believed to serve the functioning of the entire system. Adherence to gender norms could be challenging for Latinx LGBTQ people, as the intersection of their sexual and gender identity and racial and ethnic identity often defy the strict gender norms of *machismo* and *marianismo*. The role of gender norms is critical in understanding the relationship between Latinx LGBTQ people and their parents. Providers working with Latinx LGBTQ people and their families must work collaboratively to find collective goals and discuss flexible strategies to meet such goals within their unique family system. For instance, allowing Latinx parents to reflect on how gender norms influence how they parent their child may open the conversation about parenting practices that are more affirming for LGBTQ children.

Religion and spirituality are additional foundational core values in the functioning of Latinx family systems that guide interpersonal relationships (e.g., Adames &

Chavez-Duenas, 2016; Arredondo et al., 2014). For Latinx families, faith is an essential factor in building resilience and, therefore, crucial in the understanding of family relations. For instance, *fatalismo,* or the belief across Latinx culture that certain sickness and health conditions are God's will, and *personalismo,* or the emphasis on warmth, closeness, and empathy toward others (Campesino & Schwartz, 2006), are crucial in understanding the relationship between Latinx LGBTQ people and their families. The concept of accepting unplanned situations as God's will and having warmth, closeness, and empathy required to feel connected to spiritual guidance can move family members to accept and celebrate their LGBTQ family members. For instance, therapists can prompt families to consider times when unplanned events happened and the family was able to move forward through their faith in God and their connection to the family. Collectively, the understanding of Latinx family systems lies in understanding how cultural values, beliefs, and traditions guide their functioning.

4.2 Theoretical Frameworks

Because Latinx LGBTQ people's identities are multilayered, a single framework does not fully explain their experiences within the different systems that they navigate. We posit that Intersectionality Framework (Collins, 2000; Crenshaw, 1989), Latinx critical theory (LatCrit) (Valdez, 2005), and the minority stress model (Meyer, 2003, 2015) offer unique frameworks from which to holistically understand the experiences of Latinx LGBTQ people within the context of their Latinx families and communities. Through an Intersectionality Framework, this chapter considers the intersection of unique identities of Latinx LGBTQ people that cannot be explained from a singular perspective. Through this framework, we understand that Latinx LGBTQ people face both support and oppression within their family unit as a result of the interaction between their multilayered identities (e.g., Latinx, immigrants, LGBTQ) and Latinx culture's understanding of these intersecting identities. In addition, LatCrit calls for a critical understanding of how laws and policies are inherently designed to oppress and erase Latinx people in the United States. An understanding of this framework allows us to better make sense of how Latinx families grapple with the different systems that oppress them individually and collectively, and what this means for the experiences of their LGBTQ members within their family unit. Furthermore, the minority stress model suggests that LGBTQ people experience stressors that lead to negative mental health outcomes. This framework allows us to best conceptualize the individual and collective experiences of oppression that Latinx LGBTQ people experience within their family unit.

4.2.1 Intersectionality Framework

Through the lens of Intersectionality Framework (Crenshaw, 1989), we can understand some of the external complexities that impact the functioning of Latinx LGBTQ people and their families. Intersectionality Framework was developed to note the unique experiences of people based on the multiple identities they hold (Collins, 2000; Crenshaw, 1989). Specifically, intersectionality was developed to accurately understand discrimination toward Black women navigating the legal systems in the United States. According to Crenshaw (1989), oppressive systems look at particular identities while ignoring others, taking away from people's holistic and authentic experiences within different systems of oppression. Latinx LGBTQ people and their families hold multiple identities that place them at the intersection of racism, xenophobia, heterosexism, and cissexism. From an intersectionality perspective, Latinx families can be instrumental in helping their LGBTQ family members confront and cope with the different systems of oppression they navigate. For instance, family support can provide a sense of belonging that Latinx LGBTQ people need to feel empowered in the face of negative experiences within other settings (e.g., facing racism and xenophobia). Given the power of family relationships in the face of oppression and discrimination, it is critical for those who serve Latinx LGBTQ people and their families to be equipped to provide comprehensive, culturally appropriate services that both honors Latinx cultural values, beliefs, and traditions, and affirms Latinx LGBTQ people's sexual and gender identity not as separate from each other but as part of a collective experience.

4.2.2 Latinx Critical Theory

Latinx Critical Theory (LatCrit) is important to consider in understanding Latinx communities. Developed to understand the role of race and ethnicity in legal proceedings in the United States, LatCrit offers a unique lens from which to view institutional systems and the ways in which they harm Latinx communities (Valdes, 2005). For Latinx communities, the heterogeneity of their identities and experiences are erased when laws and policies insist on conceptualizing Latinx people's experiences as unidimensional, such as using broad terms like "Hispanics" or assuming that all Latinx people are cisgender and heterosexual. Therefore, one of the principal intentions of LatCrit is to give voice to the different experiences of Latinx people. To this end, it is important to not generalize the same cultural dynamics for all Latinx people. Specific to the experiences of Latinx LGBTQ people and their families, LatCrit calls for us to understand that family members have different experiences depending on their individual characteristics such as being darker skin vs. lighter skin or White, undocumented vs. documented, and LGBTQ vs. heterosexual and cisgender. Providers cannot assume that all Latinx families operate within the same rules, norms, and assumptions. Therefore, culturally sensitive interventions should place effort in learning about specific differences of each family member to best understand the interactions and functioning of the family as a collective.

4.2.3 *Minority Stress Model*

The Minority Stress Model further helps us grasp the impact of discrimination and oppression on Latinx LGBTQ people, including within their family unit. As conceptualized by the Minority Stress Model (Brooks, 1981, 1992; Meyer 2003, 2015), LGBTQ individuals experience distal stressors, or external experiences of negative occurrences (e.g., discrimination), that impact them at a proximal level, or at the internal level, as a result of negative perceptions about their sexual and/or gender identity (e.g., internalized heterosexism, fear; Brooks, 1981, 1992; Meyer 2003, 2015). From a systems perspective, if Latinx LGBTQ people are not affirmed, they cannot play their part in the family system because their cognitive and emotional capacity is being used to constantly address environmental stressors, both within and out of the family unit. For example, Latinx LGBTQ youth may experience bullying at school for their sexual orientation and/or gender identity (distal stressor), which could lead to the internalization of self-hate and/or low self-esteem. It is possible that the discomfort experienced by the child is then manifested in family dynamics (e.g., youth experiences depression and isolation from family members), which is exacerbated if family members are not supportive of their LGBTQ identity (see Abreu et al., 2022). Consequently, helping Latinx families understand the stressors that their LGBTQ family members face, as well as helping them identify resources available to increase support and acceptance of LGBTQ people, could result in increased family cohesion.

4.3 Latinx LGBTQ People and Their Families: An Overview

Latinx LGBTQ people often grapple with embracing their authentic selves while honoring their culture's values, beliefs, and traditions. In addition, family members of Latinx LGBTQ people often struggle to support their LGBTQ family members while grappling with cultural values, beliefs, and traditions that are not always inclusive of sexual and gender diversity. The importance of family has been of interest and continues to generate attention on how Latinx LGBTQ people navigate relations with their communities, such as prioritizing the needs of family members over their own. For example, in a qualitative study with 20 LGBQ Latinx people, participants expressed that *familismo* was an important cultural value that influenced their decision to disclose or conceal their sexual identity. Some participants expressed concerns about disclosing to their parents for fear that other family members would find out and disapprove or reject them (Gattamorta & Quidley-Rodriguez, 2018). In another study with 25 bisexual Latinx young adults, participants shared that their family's lack of support of their sexual identity provoked a great deal of stress, causing them to avoid conversations about their sexual identity in order to avoid disruption in the family unit. Interestingly, most participants shared that lack of family acceptance did not affect their positive regard for the family and described a strong emotional connection to their families (Muñoz-Laboy et al., 2009). It is important to note that some studies have found that when Latinx LGBT youth do not feel supported by their families, they experience negative mental health outcome such as high levels of depression and suicidality and decreased self-esteem (Abreu et al., 2022; Abreu et al., 2023b; Ryan et al., 2010).

The literature on the experiences of parental figures of LGBTQ people reports varying experiences, most commonly of psychological distress, sadness, depression, guilt, and shame when learning about their child's LGBTQ identity (see review in Abreu et al., 2019; Phillips & Ancis, 2008; Saltzburg, 2004). Specific to Latinx family members of Latinx LGBTQ people, research shows that cultural aspects such as *familismo*, gender norms, and religion and spirituality influence how Latinx families interact with their LGBTQ family members (Abreu et al., 2020a, b; Baiocco et al., 2015). For example, in a qualitative study with Latinx fathers of sexual minority children, Abreu et al. (2020a) found that Latinx fathers reported that *familismo* was a crucial aspect in choosing to accept their child's sexual identity. For instance, for Latinx fathers, making sure that their child felt part of the family was a strong motivator to accept them. Similarly, in a study by Abreu et al. (2020b), Cuban American and Puerto Rican parents of LGBTQ people reported the importance of maintaining the family unit intact as the main reason for accepting their child's sexual and gender identity. Furthermore, the role of gender norms in Latinx culture plays a crucial role in how Latinx families interact with their LGBTQ members and, ultimately, their decision to affirm and accept their sexual and/or gender identity. For example, some parents can reject the strict gender norms endorsed by their culture such as *machismo*, while others struggle to reframe these strict gender norms and express discomfort with "effeminate" or "flamboyant" behavior (Abreu et al., 2020a, b).

Religious and spiritual beliefs oftentimes lead Latinx family members to struggle to interact with their LGBTQ family members (e.g., Abreu et al., 2020a, b; Gattamorta et al., 2019). For example, in a study by Gattamorta et al. (2019), a mother reported, *"I am the mother that allowed my son to go to hell."* As we can see, religion and spirituality play a crucial role in how Latinx parental figures react to their child's LGBTQ identity. Other studies have found similar patterns about the influence of religion and spirituality in Latinx families' reaction to their LGBTQ family members, and is often a source of stress and rupture in the parent-child relationship (e.g., Abreu et al., 2020a; Ryan et al., 2010).

4.4 Implications for Resilience Practice: Culturally Sensitive Interventions

Considering the complexity of family dynamics requires a framework that helps visualize the interconnectedness of family parts that together make the whole. Based on von Bertalanffy's (von Bertalanffy & Woodger, 1933; von Bertalanffy, 1968) framework, we understand systems as a set of units that create subsystems that work together in their specific role and function to maintain the working of the entire system. Further, each subsystem is affected by the other, meaning that any changes in one subsystem affect the other; ultimately affecting the whole system's functioning. Von Bertalanffy explained that the survival of the systems depends on their openness or closeness to the environment. In families, there can be many subsystems that make up their system. For example, we can consider a family of six individuals (units) composed of various subsystems (parental figures, siblings, grandparents). A family systems framework complements intersectionality framework, LatCrit, and the minority stress model, and provides the context to understand interpersonal relationships within the family and the influence of Latinx cultural values, beliefs, and traditions in Latinx family dynamics when interacting with members of the family who identify as LGBTQ.

Culturally sensitive interventions for Latinx families have shown effective in reducing health disparities for Latinx youth (Prado et al., 2008; Santisteban et al., 2011). Furthermore, the value of attuning to cultural values when working with Latinx families has proven crucial in family therapy for Latinx communities. Emerging research has further shown the importance of considering and incorporating Latinx cultural values in working with Latinx LGBTQ people and their families (Abreu et al., 2020a, b; Lozano et al., 2022). As research continues to evolve in parenting and family functioning of Latinx LGBTQ people and their families, there is a need to consider incorporating a lens of intersectionality, the minority stress model, and LatCrit. Without a doubt, Latinx families have the resources needed to affirm and serve as a source of resilience for their LGBTQ members. Below we provide recommendations for how providers can incorporate culturally sensitive interventions with Latinx LGBTQ people and their families.

1. *Culturally Informed and Flexible Family-Based Treatment for Adolescents (CIFFTA)*: Borrowing from Structural Family Therapy (Minuchin & Nichols, 1998), Culturally Informed and Flexible Family-Based Treatment for Adolescents (CIFFTA) is an effective evidence-based intervention in working with Latinx youth and their families (Santisteban et al., 2011). In Structural Family Therapy, Minuchin speaks to the importance of recognizing the boundaries that exist within family structures. Minuchin further explains that boundaries that surround family members can be entangled or rigid, which in either extreme is what causes difficulties within family units. For instance, if the boundaries are enmeshed, Minuchin explains that members are not differentiated enough to provide their resources (such as time, energy, engagement) to the family functioning.

Likewise, rigid boundaries do not allow the influx of resources and further restrict providing resources within the family unit. Therefore, Minuchin proposed that flexible boundaries that adapt to their environment are the most likely to thrive in adverse circumstances. Through this lens, CIFFTA aims to target the process of communication patterns as critical indicators of the member's boundary, which the CIFFTA therapist targets through different culturally appropriate interventions. For instance, CIFFTA therapists are called to "block" negative interactions harmful to members, creating a new experience of positive communication patterns for the family. CIFFTA has been applied to work with Latinx LGBTQ youth and their families and has specific psychoeducational components for children and parents on gender identity and sexual orientation. For instance, therapists are encouraged to provide time for guided conversations with parents on sexual and gender identity development (Santisteban et al., 2011).

2. *Familias Unidas*. *Familias Unidas* is another evidence-based, culturally sensitive intervention to consider when working with Latinx families and youth. Developed to address the increasing health disparities of HIV and substance use in Latinx youth, Prado et al. (2008) created *Familias Unidas* to strengthen parent-child relationships by reshaping communication patterns. Like CIFFTA, *Familias Unidas* targets the structure of families by giving parents the leadership and resources to enhance parenting practices in the face of many stressors such as immigration and acculturation. A unique component of *Familias Unidas* is that parents participate in therapy group sessions with other parents, building a support system. Through these sessions, parents hear the experiences of other parents and build a network of support to evolve their parenting practices. Recent preventive science literature is growing in developing culturally sensitive family interventions for Latinx LGBTQ youth and their families. *Familias con Orgullo* (Lozano et al., 2022) was created from a series of studies actively incorporating feedback from Latinx sexual minority youth and their families. With a similar structure to *Familias Unidas*, *Familias con Orgullo* includes various levels of intervention in the family unit (e.g., youth sessions, family sessions, parent support group), with specific psychoeducation on sexual minority needs and information for parents on the LGBTQ community. For instance, specific components of psychoeducation were added as LGBTQ youth reported the need for parents to be informed about the specific needs of Latinx LGBTQ people. Additionally, communication components of the training provide parents with tools to enhance their interpersonal relationships with their LGBTQ child.
3. *Expressive Writing Interventions*. As more literature grows on the importance of parenting practices among Latinx parents of Latinx LGBTQ youth, researchers are using creative and expressive interventions. Abreu et al. (2020b) explored the Latinx cultural values (e.g., *familismo, machismo*) that play a role in parent-child relationships using writing interventions. Specifically, through journaling, Abreu et al. (2020b) asked participants to identify Latinx cultural values that present strengths and challenges in accepting their LGBTQ youth. Through this lens, researchers and practitioners have begun to use non-conventional ways to explore further how these cultural concepts inform the parenting practices of Latinx

parents of Latinx LGBTQ youth. Further understanding of the motivators behind parenting practices can aid the harnessing of cultural strengths to move Latinx LGBTQ youth and their families towards wellness within their culture. Using a writing intervention can be powerful in creating foundational understandings of feelings and emotions experienced by family members who are struggling to accept their LGBTQ child. Specifically, writing interventions may benefit those who have difficulty expressing themselves verbally. Thus, writing interventions can offer a unique way for family members of Latinx LGBTQ people to communicate and better understand each other's experiences.

4.5 Concluding Remarks

Latinx LGBTQ people are disproportionately impacted by health disparities and adverse health outcomes compared to their non-Latinx White counterparts due to societal stigma associated with their LGBTQ identity and their racial and ethnic identity (e.g., Lozano et al., 2022; Ocasio et al., 2016). As explored in this chapter, Latinx LGBTQ people hold multiple marginalized identities that make them vulnerable to multiple forms of oppression, including tension with their family members. Latinx people have a long history of experiencing structural, relational, and personal discrimination in the United States (see review in Adames & Chavez-Dueñas, 2016). From enforcement of anti-immigrant policies to the passing of anti-LGBTQ bills, Latinx LGBTQ people and their families are positioned within multiple forms of oppression, including racism, homophobia, heterosexism, ethnocentrism, and nativism. Thus, the authors suggest that clinicians commit to understanding the ways in which oppression impacts the interaction between Latinx LGBTQ people and their families. Specifically, we posit that clinicians must learn about different Latinx cultural values, beliefs, and traditions, as well as about different frameworks that contextualize how Latinx LGBTQ people experience privilege and oppression, before implementing interventions that may ultimately harm or inaccurately address the presenting concerns of Latinx LGBTQ people and their families. Finally, although researchers and clinicians have been slow to develop interventions that address the intersectional needs of Latinx LGBTQ people within the context of their families and communities, CIFFTA, *Familias Unidas*, and expressive writing interventions have been successful in working with Latinx LGBTQ people and their families.

Questions for Thought and Discussion

1. How can practitioners who work with Latinx LGBTQ people and their families incorporate frameworks of intersectionality, LatCrit, and minority stress in conceptualizing these communities' presenting concerns?
2. What is the importance of understanding and incorporating Latinx cultural values, beliefs, and traditions in working with Latinx LGBTQ people and their families?

3. Which aspects of the culturally sensitive interventions outlined in this chapter (i.e., CIFFTA, *Familias Unidas*, and expressive writing), do you find most valuable in working Latinx LGBTQ people and their families?

Conflicts of Interests We have no conflicts of interests to disclose

References

Abreu, R. L., Rosenkrantz, D. E., Ryser-Oatman, J. T., Rostosky, S. S., & Riggle, E. D. (2019). Parental reactions to transgender and gender diverse children: A literature review. *Journal of GLBT Family Studies, 15*(5), 461–485. https://doi.org/10.1080/1550428X.2019.1656132

Abreu, R. L., Gonzalez, K. A., Rosario, C. C., Pulice-Farrow, L., & Rodríguez, M. M. D. (2020a). "Latinos have a stronger attachment to the family": Latinx fathers' acceptance of their sexual minority children. *Journal of GLBT Family Studies, 16*(2), 192–210. https://doi.org/10.1080/1550428X.2019.1672232

Abreu, R. L., Riggle, E. D., & Rostosky, S. S. (2020b). Expressive writing intervention with Cuban-American and Puerto Rican parents of LGBTQ individuals. *The Counseling Psychologist, 48*(1), 106–134. https://doi.org/10.1177/0011000019853240

Abreu, R. L., Lefevor, G. T., Gonzalez, K. A., Barrita, A. M., & Watson, R. J. (2022). Bullying, depression, and parental acceptance in a sample of Latinx sexual and gender minority youth. *Journal of LGBT Youth*, 1–18. Advance online publication. https://doi.org/10.1080/19361653.2022.2071791.

Abreu, R. L., Barrita, A. M., Martin, J. A., Sostre, J., & Gonzalez, K. A. (2023a). Latinx LGBTQ youth, COVID-19, and psychological well-being: A systematic review. *Journal of Clinical Child & Adolescent Psychology.* Online First. https://doi.org/10.1080/15374416.2022.2158839

Abreu, R. L., Skidmore, S. J., Badio, K. S., Lefevor, G. T., Gattamorta, K. A., & Watson, R. J. (2023b). Sexual harassment, sexual assault, violence, self-esteem, and the role of LGBTQ-specific parental support in a sample of Latinx sexual and gender minority youth. *Journal of Adolescence.* Online First. https://doi.org/10.1002/jad.12210

Adames, H. Y., & Chavez-Dueñas, N. Y. (2016). *Cultural foundations and interventions in Latino/a mental health: History, theory and within group differences.* Routledge. https://doi.org/10.4324/9781315724058

Arredondo, P., Gallardo-Cooper, M., Delgado-Romero, E. A., & Zapata, A. L. (2014). *Culturally responsive counseling with Latinas/os*. Wiley.

Baiocco, R., Fontanesi, L., Santamaria, F., Ioverno, S., Marasco, B., Baumgartner, E., Willoughby, B. L., & Laghi, F. (2015). Negative parental responses to coming out and family functioning in a sample of lesbian and gay young adults. *Journal of Child and Family Studies, 24*(5), 1490–1500. https://doi.org/10.1007/s10826-014-9954-z

Bostwick, W. B., Meyer, I., Aranda, F., Russell, S., Hughes, T., Birkett, M., & Mustanski, B. (2014). Mental health and suicidality among racially/ethnically diverse sexual minority youths. *American Journal of Public Health, 104*(6), 1129–1136. https://doi.org/10.2105/AJPH.2013.301749

Brooks, V. R. (1981). *Minority stress and lesbian women.* Free Press.

Brooks, W. K. (1992). Research and the gay minority: Problems and possibilities. In N. J. Woodman (Ed.), *Lesbian and gay lifestyles: A guide for counseling and education* (pp. 201–215). Irvington.

Campesino, M., & Schwartz, G. E. (2006). Spirituality among Latinas/os: Implications of culture in conceptualization and measurement. *Advances in Nursing Science, 29*(1), 69–81. https://doi.org/10.1097/00012272-200601000-00007

Collins, P. H. (2000). *Black feminist thought: Knowledge, consciousness, and the politics of empowerment*. Patricia Hill Collins.

Cortés-García, L., Hernandez Ortiz, J., Asim, N., Sales, M., Villareal, R., Penner, F., & Sharp, C. (2022). COVID-19 conversations: A qualitative study of majority Hispanic/Latinx youth experiences during early stages of the pandemic. *Child & Youth Care Forum, 51*, 769–793. https://doi.org/10.1007/s10566-021-09653-x

Costa, S., Rodriguez, A., Grant, S., Hernandez, M., Alvarez Bautista, J., Houchin, Q., Brown, A., & Calcagno, A. (2021). Outcomes of COVID-19 on Latinx youth: Considering the role of adverse childhood events and resilience. *School Psychology, 36*(5), 335–347. https://doi.org/10.1037/spq0000459

Crenshaw, K. (1989). Demarginalizing the intersection of race and sex: A black feminist critique of antidiscrimination doctrine, feminist theory and antiracist politics. *University of Chicago Legal Forum, 1989*(1), 139–167.

Gattamorta, K., & Quidley-Rodriguez, N. (2018). Coming out experiences of Hispanic sexual minority young adults in South Florida. *Journal of Homosexuality, 65*(6), 741–765. https://doi.org/10.1080/00918369.2017.1364111

Gattamorta, K. A., Salerno, J., & Quidley-Rodriguez, N. (2019). Hispanic parental experiences of learning a child identifies as a sexual minority. *Journal of GLBT Family Studies, 15*(2), 151–164. https://doi.org/10.1080/1550428X.2018.1518740

Gil, R. M., & Vazquez, C. I. (1996). *The maria paradox: How Latinas can merge old world traditions with new world self-esteem*. G. P. Putnam's Sons.

Harkness, A., Behar-Zusman, V., & Safren, S. A. (2020). Understanding the impact of COVID-19 on Latino sexual minority men in a US HIV hot spot. *AIDS and Behavior, 24*(7), 2017–2023.

Kann, L., McManus, T., Harris, W. A., Shanklin, S. L., Flint, K. H., Queen, B., Lowry, R., Chyen, D., Whittle, L., Thornton, J., Lim, C., Bradford, D., Yamakawa, Y., Leon, M., Brener, N., & Ethier, K. A. (2018). Youth risk behavior surveillance – United States, 2017. *Morbidity and Mortality Weekly Report. Surveillance Summaries, 67*(8), 1–114. https://doi.org/10.15585/mmwr.ss6708a1

Lozano, A., Estrada, Y., Tapia, M. I., Dave, D. J., Marquez, N., Baudin, S., & Prado, G. (2022). Development of a family-based preventive intervention for Latinx sexual minority youth and their parents. *Cultural Diversity and Ethnic Minority Psychology, 28*(2), 227–239. https://doi.org/10.1037/cdp0000506

Manzano-Sanchez, H., Matarrita-Cascante, D., & Outley, C. (2019). Barriers and supports to college aspiration among Latinx high school students. *Journal of Youth Development, 14*(2), 25–45. https://doi.org/10.5195/jyd.2019.685

Marin, G., & Marin, B. V. (1991). *Research with Hispanic populations*. Sage.

Mayo, Y. (1997). Machismo, fatherhood and the Latino family: Understanding the concept. *Journal of Multicultural Social Work, 5*(1–2), 49–61. https://doi.org/10.1300/J285v05n01_05

Meyer, I. H. (2003). Prejudice, social stress, and mental health in lesbian, gay, and bisexual populations: Conceptual issues and research evidence. *Psychological Bulletin, 129*(5), 674–697. https://doi.org/10.1037/00332909.129.5.674

Meyer, I. H. (2015). Resilience in the study of minority stress and health of sexual and gender minorities. *Psychology of Sexual Orientation and Gender Diversity, 2*(3), 209–213. https://doi.org/10.1037/sgd0000132

Minuchin, S., & Nichols, M. P. (1998). Structural family therapy. In F. M. Dattilio (Ed.), *Case studies in couple and family therapy: Systemic and cognitive perspectives* (pp. 108–131). Guilford Press.

Muñoz-Laboy, M., Leau, C. J. Y., Sriram, V., Weinstein, H. J., del Aquila, E. V., & Parker, R. (2009). Bisexual desire and familism: Latino/a bisexual young men and women in New York City. *Culture, Health & Sexuality, 11*(3), 331–344. https://doi.org/10.1080/13691050802710634

Needham, B. L., & Austin, E. L. (2010). Sexual orientation, parental support, and health during the transition to young adulthood. *Journal of Youth and Adolescence, 39*(10), 1189–1198. https://doi.org/10.1007/s10964-010-9533-6

Ocasio, M. A., Feaster, D. J., & Prado, G. (2016). Substance use and sexual risk behavior in sexual minority Hispanic adolescents. *Journal of Adolescent Health, 59*(5), 599–601. https://doi.org/10.1016/j.jadohealth.2016.07.008

Penner, F., Ortiz, J. H., & Sharp, C. (2021). Change in youth mental health during the COVID-19 pandemic in a majority Hispanic/Latinx US sample. *Journal of the American Academy of Child & Adolescent Psychiatry, 60*(4), 513–523. https://doi.org/10.1016/j.jaac.2020.12.027

Phillips, M. J., & Ancis, J. R. (2008). The process of identity development as the parent of a lesbian or gay male. *Journal of LGBT Issues in Counseling, 2*(2), 126–158. https://doi.org/10.1080/15538600802125605

Prado, G., Szapocznik, J., Maldonado-Molina, M. M., Schwartz, S. J., & Pantin, H. (2008). Drug use/abuse prevalence, etiology, prevention, and treatment in Hispanic adolescents: A cultural perspective. *Journal of Drug Issues, 38*(1), 5–36. https://doi.org/10.1177/002204260803800010

Ryan, C., Russell, S. T., Huebner, D., Diaz, R., & Sanchez, J. (2010). Family acceptance in adolescence and the health of LGBT young adults. *Journal of Child and Adolescent Psychiatric Nursing, 23*(4), 205–213. https://doi.org/10.1111/j.1744-6171.2010.00246.x

Saewyc, E. M., Homma, Y., Skay, C. L., Bearinger, L. H., Resnick, M. D., & Reis, E. (2009). Protective factors in the lives of bisexual adolescents in North America. *American Journal of Public Health, 99*(1), 110–117.

Saez, P. A., Casado, A., & Wade, J. C. (2010). Factors influencing masculinity ideology among Latino men. *The Journal of Men's Studies, 17*(2), 116–128. https://doi.org/10.3149/jms.1702.11

Saltzburg, S. (2004). Learning that an adolescent child is gay or lesbian: The parent experience. *Social Work, 49*(1), 109–118. https://doi.org/10.1093/sw/49.1.109

Santisteban, D. A., Mena, M. P., & McCabe, B. E. (2011). Preliminary results for an adaptive family treatment for drug abuse in Hispanic youth. *Journal of Family Psychology, 25*(4), 610. https://doi.org/10.1037/a0024016

Valdes, F. (2005). Legal reform and social justice: An introduction to LatCrit theory, praxis and community. *Griffith Law Review, 14*(2), 148–173. https://doi.org/10.1080/10383441.2005.10854554

Victor, A., Zaman, F., Cho, M., & Callejas, P. (2020). Latinx immigrants' healthcare access: Barriers, consequences and strategies for the future. *Undergraduate Research Posters. Poster 335*. https://scholarscompass.vcu.edu/uresposters/335

von Bertalanffy, L. (1968). *General systems theory: Foundation development and application*. George Braziller.

von Bertalanffy, L., & Woodger, J. H. (1933). *Modern theories of development: An introduction to theoretical biology* (Vol. 554). Oxford University Press.

Chapter 5
I'm *That* Girl: Promoting Resilience and Reclaiming Black Girl Voice

Sheretta T. Butler-Barnes

Black girls in today's society face racism and sexism in educational settings (Blake et al., 2011; Butler-Barnes et al., 2022; Carter Andrews et al., 2019; Rogers & Butler-Barnes, 2021). Racism is the root cause of both prejudice and discrimination, which can be defined as the formation of unfavorable attitudes or beliefs regarding members of other racial groups, and the discriminating treatment of members of these groups by both people and societal institutions (Williams & Mohammed, 2009). Sexism is a form of prejudice or discrimination that is founded on misconceptions about a person's sex or gender (Mills, 2016). Due to their racialized and gendered experiences, Black girls face both racism and sexism. Because of Black girls' racialized and gendered experiences, they contend with both – racism and sexism.

Butler-Barnes et al. (2022), for example, found that Black girls' perceptions of gender and racial discrimination from teachers were associated with increased suicide ideation. Teachers were also more likely to view Black girls as unintelligent (Carter-Andrews et al., 2019). These findings indicate how racism and sexism contribute to negative perceptions and biases toward Black girls. This study expands our understanding of the within-group variability of Black girls and how they interpret their educational environment. This study examines a sample of Black girls from several school districts in a Midwestern metropolis. These distinct school districts include schools that are mainly White, schools that are predominantly Black, schools that are racially and ethnically diverse, private schools, and charter schools. It is important to understand Black girls' experiences in a variety of contexts and how they navigate racism and sexism. Overall, the purpose of the study was to understand Black girls' experiences in context and the resilient coping strategies

S. T. Butler-Barnes (✉)
Washington University in St. Louis, St. Louis, MO, USA
e-mail: sbarnes22@wustl.edu

J. M. Koch et al. (eds.), *Identity as Resilience in Minoritized Communities*, Emerging Issues in Family and Individual Resilience,
https://doi.org/10.1007/978-3-031-38977-1_5

they used to deal with stressors due to their racialized and gendered status within the school context.

Since the nineteenth century, Black girls have had to contend with racism and misogynoir (e.g., the intersection of racism & sexism that produces racialized gendered violence) (Simmons, 2015, Wright, 2016). This includes but is not limited to Black girls being hypersexualized and perceived as angry, promiscuous, sassy, ghetto, and loud (Morris, 2007). In addition to these negative stereotypes, there is burgeoning literature that has documented the negative impact of stereotypes and impact on learning. These investigations range from their experiences in STEM (Science, Technology, Engineering, & Mathematics) classrooms (Ibrahim et al., 2021) to their interactions with classroom teachers (Butler-Barnes et al., 2021). In addition to these experiences, there is research literature that documents the extent to which Black girls are overdisciplined and harassed in school settings (Blake et al., 2011, 2022; Epstein et al., 2017; Morris, 2016), and how these negative racialized and gendered experiences lead to higher suspension and expulsion rates. For instance, Blake et al. (2022) found that Black girls were more likely to be disciplined based on teacher's philosophy on discipline and teacher's racial and ethnic background. Similarly, Blake et al. (2011) found that Black girls were overrepresented in exclusionary school discipline in comparison to their White and Hispanic peers.

The challenges Black girls face have their origins in entrenched forms of racism and sexism. For instance, in the nineteenth century, the late Sojourner Truth spoke about the injustices against Black women. Specifically, Truth emphasized that Black women's work was continuously disregarded and undervalued in that era's culture. As a result, we are now well into the twenty-first century, and a plethora of research indicates that Black girls continue to face challenges in larger environments that place them at risk for harmful educational experiences and poor overall health and well-being (Butler- Barnes et al., 2022; Stokes et al., 2020).

Further, there is burgeoning literature indicating that experiences that Black girls face on a daily basis as a result of the intersection of their social identities might be associated with poorer mental health outcomes (Butler-Barnes et al., 2022; Stokes et al., 2020). In a study conducted by Butler-Barnes et al. (2022), the findings revealed that Black girls who experienced higher levels of racial and gender discrimination from their teachers were more likely to report higher depressive symptoms. Black girls in this study were similarly more likely to report higher rates of suicidal ideation when exposed to greater levels of racial and gender discrimination. It is also important to note that there are major reports, such as the *Let Her Learn: Unlocking the Opportunity for Black Girls*, and the Georgetown Law Poverty Center's *The Erasure of Black Girlhood* reports (Epstein et al., 2017; Onyeka-Crawford et al., 2017; Smith-Evans et al., 2014), that highlight the lived experiences of Black girls and the impact of racism and sexism on their well-being and social mobility. Consequently, the current study contributes to the scholarly literature by shedding light on the lived experiences of Black girls.

More specifically, this study contributes to the literature by expanding our understanding of the within-group variability of Black girls and how they interpret their educational environment. This study examines a sample of Black girls from several school districts in a Midwestern metropolis. These distinct school districts include schools that are mainly White, schools that are predominantly Black, schools that are racially and ethnically diverse, private schools, and charter schools. It is important to understand Black girls' experiences in a variety of contexts and how they navigate racism and sexism. There was also interest in the social support systems that Black girls identified as a means of coping with negative experiences in the school setting. In this approach, it is not merely naming the experiences of Black girls in context; rather, the centering of their voices is imperative to inform us about the support structures that allow them to thrive inside the school setting. Thus, this work contributes to the body of knowledge in a number of ways. First, it broadens our present understanding of Black girls, as they are not a monolith. Second, because of the dearth of research on the experiences of Black girls in diverse school settings, no immediate hypotheses were formulated concerning their experiences. In the studies that have explored the experiences of Black girls, teachers perceive them to be less intellectual, have lower expectations for their performance, and are more likely to penalize them than White girls in schools where the majority of students are White (Carter Andrews et al., 2019). In addition to these negative experiences, Black girls must contend with White femininity and norms, which are destructive to their identity and the way they define what it means to be a Black girl (Esposito & Edwards, 2018). This study expands this line of inquiry by centering the experiences of Black girls in a meaningful way and by seeking to understand their lived experiences in diverse educational environments.

5.1 Black Girls in School Settings

Several studies in the academic literature document the lived experiences of Black girls in school settings. Because of the unique social positioning of Black girls, they often have to contend with racism, sexism, and classism. In this study, I use intersectionality (Crenshaw, 1989, 1995) as a guide to understand Black girls' lived experiences within the school context. Intersectionality is the intersection of race, gender, and socioeconomic status, and Black girls face multiple forms of oppression and marginalization (Crenshaw, 1989, 1995). Thus, it is important to discuss the scholarship that has contributed to our knowing of how Black girls have been treated in school settings. For instance, majority of the research literature that has examined Black girls in school settings has found that teachers generally have lower expectations for them; their teachers are more likely to view them as sassy; their teachers are more likely to compare them to White femininity and standards; and Black girls are more likely to be overdisciplined and suspended (Blake et al., 2011, 2022; Carter Andrews et al., 2019; Morris, 2007, 2016). According to Epstein et al. (2017), Black girls were more likely than their non-Black counterparts to be suspended for dress and minor offenses. *Girlhood Interrupted: The Erasure of Black Girls' Childhood* (Epstein et al., 2017) report found that adults in their study perceived Black girls as needing less nurturing, needing less protection, needing to be supported less, and needing to be comforted less. Black girls also were perceived to be more independent, knowing more about adult topics, and to know more about sex. Black girls also spoke about the negative teacher-student relationships and their bodies being policed (Nunn, 2018). Corroborating previous literature, Black girls were also compared with White femininity standards, loaded up with negative stereotypes, and to be viewed as unintelligent (Nunn, 2018). In predominately White school spaces, Black girls also perceived lower academic expectations from teachers (Butler et al., 2019a, b).

Further, the suspension of Black girls might have a negative effect on their ability to matriculate in their learning environment. For instance, Ibrahim et al. (2021) found that among a nationally representative sample of Black girls, in-school suspension was associated with being less likely to be on a STEM pathway. Consequently, Black girls' being suspended, whether in-school or out-of-school, have devastating implications on their learning. Other literature has noted that teachers' inequitable demands are damaging to the well-being and identity of Black girls. For instance, Carter Andrews et al. (2019) examined a sample of Black girls who attended a predominantly White school and found that Black girls frequently have to contend with the stereotypes and biases of teachers who compared them to White girls which resulted in them being more likely to feel ostracized, isolated, and to feel as if they didn't belong. In addition to having a negative effect on their well-being, the racism and sexism that surrounds Black girls in school settings is also damaging to their mental health (Butler-Barnes et al., 2022; Stokes et al. 2020). As previously noted, Black girls who perceive both racial and gender discrimination reported higher levels of depressive symptoms and suicidal ideation (Butler-Barnes et al., 2022). In other studies, Chavous et al. (2008) found that racial discrimination was related to lower levels of school importance among Black girls.

Moreover, a number of research studies have identified factors that promote the success of Black girls in educational spaces. For instance, the studies that have centered Black girls have explored the relationship between racial pride and their academic attitudes and beliefs. For example, Butler-Barnes et al. (2018) found that Black girls who expressed higher levels of racial pride over time demonstrated more academic curiosity. In the same study, Black girls also stated that a sense of belonging within the school was associated with higher academic beliefs and attitudes such as academic persistence and academic curiosity. Thus, in school settings where Black girls are permitted to be themselves and where they are encouraged, they are more likely to have a sense of belonging and to express a higher level of intellectual curiosity. In an effort to advance this work, we strive to understand the meaning-making of Black girls in a variety of educational settings and their experiences. Often, we recognize that racism and sexism effect Black girls in ways that are distinctive from those of other racial and ethnic minority groups, but it's also crucial to notice for Black girls the settings that influence their learning and well-being. Thus, the purpose of this exploratory study is to gain an understanding of what Black girls' school experiences and relationships with teachers and peers are like. And do they feel like they belong in their particular school setting? Because the questions are open-ended, the findings will contribute to the existing research by gaining a better knowledge of how Black girls deal with racism and sexism in school.

5.1.1 Resistance and Resilience

This concept of resistance and resilience is based on earlier research that has shown Black girls are also capable of rejecting the negative stereotypes and ideas held by our community (Kelly, 2018, 2020; Rogers et al., 2021). For instance, one of the ways that contemporary research literature has documented the resilience of Black girls despite their unfavorable classroom experiences due to racism and sexism is through the hashtag *Black girl magic*. In the study conducted by Rogers et al. (2021) the findings revealed that the #Blackgirlmagic is important for Black girls, as it reinforced who they were and allowed them to redefine, reclaim, and defy the daily negative stereotypes they face. In another study, Rogers and Butler-Barnes (2021) found that Black girls within a predominately Black all-girl school noted that access to resources would help them thrive and perform well academically. This is particularly significant since it demonstrates that Black girls are not merely passive in the classroom but are knowers of what is beneficial for them and what would impact their social mobility.

In this study, I seek to contribute to the research literature by understanding the ways in which not only Black girls experience the context, but also the deliberate and intentional ways in which Black girls are resisting and reclaiming their voices, while also combating racism, sexism, and classism in schools.

5.1.2 Guiding Framework

Black girls have unique gendered and racialized statuses. It is critical to look at how schools influence Black girls' developmental abilities since they must deal with racist tropes and stereotypes (Carter-Andrews et al., 2019; Morris, 2007). In this study, we use Black Feminist Theory (BFT), an intersectional framework, to analyze how Black girls succeed in academic environments where they are perceived as "less than" because of their race and gender identities (Collins, 2000). By concentrating on race or gender separately, Black girls' experiences in the classroom are frequently unreported, misunderstood, or completely disregarded. BFT encourages scholars to go beyond summarizing Black girls' experiences as students and instead focus on developing anti-racist and anti-sexist solutions that will end the continued marginalization of these girls. The Integrative Model for the Developmental Competencies of Minority Children is another framework that is drawn upon (Garcia-Coll et al., 1996). It's crucial to consider how one's social position status (race/ethnicity, class, and gender) plays a specific function in shaping experiences in a school environment. According to Coll et al. (1996), the school atmosphere can either be a place that fosters learning or a place that discourages it. Positive developmental outcomes are produced as a result of positive circumstances that support positive developmental competencies. Negative developmental consequences are caused by inhibiting factors. Self-esteem, academic success, mental wellness, psychological well-being, and identity are just a few examples of developmental competencies. The social positioning (race, ethnicity, class, and gender) of Black youth matters since classrooms can be encouraging or discouraging spaces, thus we extend this study by emphasizing the voices of Black girls. By referencing Black feminist theory, how much do varied classroom environments affect how Black girls perceive themselves and how that affects their well-being? By focusing on Black girls in various racial, cultural, and socioeconomically diverse educational environments, our study expands on this body of work. This study contributes to the body of knowledge already available about the space that Black girls occupy because they are not a homogeneous group. Collectively, we were interested in the ways that particular environments affect Black girls' wellness, attitudes toward and ideas about academics, and overall experiences, noticing both the parallels and disparities in the environments they occupy. More importantly, we want to comprehend their school-related experiences. These queries were posed to Black girls: (1) Describe the atmosphere at your school; (2) How are you treated by your teachers at school?; and (3) How would you describe your experiences at school?

5.2 Positionality Statement

I identify as an African American woman from a middle-class environment who attended a predominantly Black school and grew up in the inner city. The fact that I attended a primarily Black school at the time insulated me in some ways from experiencing a highly racialized setting; nonetheless, it is crucial to emphasize that I did suffer sexism in these educational spaces. My work as a scholar has compelled me to pay special attention to the needs of Black girls in this area in order to truly explore and comprehend their lived experiences. The research team members attended a variety of school settings: predominantly Black schools, racially and ethnically diverse schools, private schools, and charter schools. Consequently, the research team reflected both the population in which we were interested and the population which we sought to serve. We approach this project by valuing the voices of Black girls. Centering Black girls' experiences and allowing them to express their stories is necessary for conducting equitable research with them, limiting our misinterpretations, misrepresentations, and acquisition of false information about Black girls (see Milner, 2007). Our racial, gender, and social class backgrounds let us go around the educational environment and actively listen to the stories of Black females.

5.3 Methods

To investigate Black girls' experiences at their school, we employed an inductive, qualitative study design (Creswell, 2012). Focus groups were held with a sample of Black girls in sixth through ninth grades from a variety of educational environments. Due to an existing connection the principal investigator (first author) has with the participating school districts, recruiting was made easier. In order to better comprehend Black girl space, we recruited students from a variety of educational institutions, including those who attended private and public schools with a range of socioeconomic, racial, and ethnic make-up.

We were all interested in comprehending the many encounters that Black girls had in these various contexts. Flyers were circulated to local schools to encourage Black girls to enroll in the study. A snowball sampling strategy was also used to bring in more kids from the school. Parents who were interested in participating returned signed forms after receiving student information packets at home. After contacting the parents, the study's primary investigator went over the study's details and addressed any queries or worries they may have had about their child taking part. Parental permission to speak with their adolescent personally and consent for their child to participate in the study were gained verbally. Three Black women from the data collection team—a developmental psychologist and two MSW graduate students—called students to describe the study and get their verbal consent to participate. Seven people made up the research team, including the aforementioned data gatherers and three additional analysts.

5.3.1 *Participants*

The average age of the 30 Black girls that took part in the study was 12.64. Parents often reported having some college experience, and the majority were married. The participant's parents had an average yearly salary of between $40,000 and $49,000. Black girls were chosen for the program from a variety of racial and cultural schools (see Table 5.1). Sixteen girls were from predominately White school districts, eight Black girls from predominately Black school districts, and six Black girls from racially and ethnically diverse school districts. Pseudonyms were used (see Table 5.2).

5.3.2 *Data Collection*

We held four focus groups with a total of 30 Black adolescent girls, with an average of 6 to 8 females per session. The sessions were scheduled in accordance with the girls' extracurricular and school schedules. The discussion of girls' racialized and

Table 5.1 School demographics

	# of Students	Black	American Indian	Latinx	White	Other	Asian	Multiracial
Predominately white schools								
Sledge middle school (public)	8	2%	1%	0%	80%	0%	13%	1%
Poppins middle school (public)	7	2.2%	0%	0.6%	92%	1%	3.9%	0%
Montessori school (private)	1	5%	1%	2%	66%	1%	13%	15%
Predominately black schools								
Hillman middle school (public)	1	99%	0%	0%	0%	0%	0%	1%
Scholar middle school (public)	1	99%	0%	0%	0%	1%	0%	0%
Jefferson middle school (charter)	6	98%	0%	0%	0%	0%	0%	2%
Racially & ethnically diverse schools								
Hope middle school (public)	4	27.1%	0%	3.4%	64.4%	0%	1.6%	3.4%
Warner middle school (public)	2	43.5%	1%	15.4%	32.8%	0%	2.2%	5.5%

Note: Number of students that participating in the study from the specific school. The racial ethnic composition of the participating school is noted. Other is comprised of American Indian and Pacific Islander

Table 5.2 Participant demographics

Participant name	Age	Family income	Parent educational level	School setting
Janae	14.34	\$30,000–\$39,999	High school diploma	PWS
Layla	14.15	\$50,000–\$59,999	Some graduate school	PWS
Kendall	14.34	\$30,000–\$39,999	High school diploma	PWS
Ke'era	13.01	\$20,000–\$29,999	Some college	PBS
Zoe	13.24	\$30,000–\$39,999	High school diploma	PBS
Tekise	13.49	\$30,000–\$39,999	Master's degree	PWS
Monique	12.96	\$70,000–\$79,999	Master's degree	PWS
Sia	13.39	\$20,000–\$29,999	Some graduate school	PWS
Nikia	12.51	\$10,000–\$19,999	College diploma	PWS
Jayla	12.53	\$60,000–\$69,999	Some college	PBS
Tia	12.72	\$30,000–\$39,999	Some college	PBS
Summer	13.37	\$80,000–\$89,999	College diploma	PWS
Aaliyah	13.90	Less than \$10,000	Some high school	PWS
Rihanna	14.42	\$30,000–\$39,999	College diploma	PWS
Nicole	13.46	\$30,000–\$39,999	College diploma	RED

Note: *PWS* Predominately white schools, *PBS* Predominately black schools, and *RED* Racially and ethnically diverse schools gendered experiences in the classroom was sparked by the use of semi-structured focus group guides. To better understand the impact that race and gender had on their educational experiences, we asked specific questions on how they interacted with their teachers and peers. Each focus group was scheduled outside of school hours and held at the local institution. Focus groups were not established by students from one particular school due to the small number of students recruited and to varying student schedules (see Table 5.1). A member of the research team discussed confidentiality and acquired written consent from each participant (each teenager and parent) prior to each adolescent's arrival at the institution. After the focus group interviews, which lasted around 1.5 h per focus group, participants were given a $20.00 gift card from Barnes & Noble bookstores.

5.3.3 Coding Analysis

After gathering the data, the transcription of the audio recordings was contracted out. The study team, which was made up of three Black women—a developmental psychologist and two MSW graduate students—verified the focus groups' verbatim transcripts to ensure correctness, particularly with regard to language and dialect that might have been omitted or transcribed improperly. To accurately capture how Black girls report their school experiences, the verification procedure is essential. The focus group transcripts were then entered into Atlas.ti, a platform for analyzing qualitative data (Scientific Software Development Company, 2011). Data analysis methods based on grounded theory (such as constant comparisons, coding, etc.) were utilized in order to explore conversational trends (Charmaz, 2002; Strauss & Corbin, 1998).

To help in coding the transcripts, four more students were enlisted. Thus, over the course of the Fall 2016 semester, six graduate research assistants and the P.I. met on a weekly basis to create emergent codes and topics. Each transcript was read by the study team. Each transcript was about 100 pages long. Each transcript was classified separately by the research team, who used open coding to look for beginning categories and codes. Following individual coding, the study team gathered to discuss the initial codes and categories that had developed. We addressed our individual initial interpretations of what Black girls were talking about at their school during this discussion. The research team collaborated to define each code during weekly meetings held throughout the academic semester in order to generate numerous iterations of codes derived from the data. Each member of the study team looked at each transcript separately while using these analytical questions as a guide to find emerging codes. The study team's definitions were considered, and codes were developed. Our first meeting's initial coding of themes served as the basis for subsequent meetings' revisions and creation of new codes. Then, we created a number of iterations. The research teams reread each transcript and convened to discuss any disagreements after evaluating and checking the whole list of codes and meanings. There was 85% agreement overall. The coding of the definitions was the

Table 5.3 Demographics characteristics cont'd

Participant name	Age	Family income	Parent educational level	School setting
Rasheeda	12.23	$80,000–$89,999	PhD/MD/JD	PWS
Kristen	12.45	$80,000–$89,999	PhD/MD/JD	RED
Taraji	12.96	$80,000–$89,999	PhD/MD/JD	PWS
Kimora	11.75	$30,000–$39,999	Some graduate school	PBS
Sanaa	14.46	$60,000–$69,999	Master's degree	RED
Ke'era	14.27	$30,000–$39,999	College diploma	PWS

cause of 15% of the discrepancies. These codes were subsequently recoded in order to gain consensus within the study team. After every meeting, codes were produced. The study team met to talk definitions over and come to an agreement as new codes appeared. When necessary, codes and meanings were changed to represent the participants' voices more precisely (see Table 5.3.)

5.4 Results: Resistance, Reclaiming, and Resilience

In this study, Black girls discussed their diverse school experiences. Black girls discussed the strategies and support they use to reclaim their sense of self and to resist negative treatment and stereotypes. These experiences varied by school type. This study's findings corroborate previous research citing Black girls' mistreatment and invisibility in the classroom (Butler-Barnes et al., 2018; Carter Andrews et al., 2019; Nunn, 2018).

5.4.1 Resistance: I Know Who I Am

Black girls reported being unheard, unseen, and undervalued with regard to their intellectual capacity and sense of self. More specifically, Black girls shared stories, highlighting the similarities and differences within each of the educational spaces. Black girls, despite their experiences in these school settings, emphasized the importance of space and sisterhood as they navigated racist and sexist school environments, while also being intentional standing strong in the face of injustice (Table 5.4).

Tekise: To be honest, like Black people get called different names than White people. But it – so it's all just playing around. It's not like it really means anything. You know, they just toss it around.

Nia: But it does mean something, because if somebody says that to a Black person, they're going to go and like say it to somebody else, and that's going to start a bigger problem.

Kimora: And it's just – it's just offensive, because they'll call-say it because you are Black, but they won't say it to a White person.

Table 5.4 Participant demographics characteristics cont'd

Participant name	Age	Family income	Parent educational level	School setting
Hannah	13.83	$30,000–$39,999	College Diploma	RED
Simone	10.08	$20,000–$29,999	Some graduate school	PWS
Parker	12.61	$10,000–$19,999	College diploma	RED
Akelee	12.62	$40,000–$49,999	Some graduate school	PWS
Tasha	13.52	$40,000–$49,999	College diploma	PBS
Jamiya	12.06	$40,000–$49,999	Some graduate school	PBS
Makayla	12.08	$40,000–$49,999	Some college	PBS
Aaliyah	12.31	$50,000–$59,999	Master's degree	PWS
Nia	12.54	$30,000–$39,999	Some college	RED

Note: *PWS* Predominately white schools, *PBS* Predominately black schools, and *RED* Racially and ethnically diverse schools

> Monique*:* At our school, it's like a little difference, like the fact if you – if a White person – a White person called you a name, then you would want to go to the principal and say something. The principal and assistant principal are White, so what's the point of going to them when they're probably won't – like whether or not – it's like a uh, like defend you or say what you want them to really say. So it's no point of going to them, just defend yourself, and wherever it goes, at least you, uh, stood proud for what you believed in.

Black girls are discussing the negative experiences they encounter at school in this conversation. These conversations occurred primarily among Black girls who attended schools that were predominantly White and, in some cases, racially and ethnically diverse. Black girls discussed how they knew the way they were treated was unjust, but also how little, if anything, can be done to address the issue. For example, Monique asserts that it is pointless to speak with the principal or vice principal because they are White. However, she emphasized the significance of defending herself and standing proud. I then probed further to understand why Monique felt as if the administration (e.g., principal, vice principal, or those in charge) would not support her. Monique states the following:

> I could have went to the principal. But, it's a mostly White school, it's no point of doing it. They might not be racist. They might be. But I – I just didn't go. If I heard it again, keep doing what I have to do, and let it get, um, higher in the, uh, administrative area (school district level). Then others can hear…like the preachers and we can stay strong, stuff like that. People can really hear what's going on, and like just more people come out and do another march, because I'll do as many marches as it takes to, uh, get our race, you know, to stand proud.

In this particular school district, there was some unrest after the death of Michael Brown and Monique noted how on a daily basis, Black students had to defend themselves and participate in walk-outs to be heard. In this instance, Monique is discussing how to remain strong and how to involve others from the community.

5.4.2 *Reclaiming: Racial Pride*

Despite the negative encounters in schools, Black girls talked about how proud they were despite the negative treatment and the importance of Black history and the accomplishments of Black Americans. Examples of Black history and the struggle and resilience of Black people gave Black girls hope so they could persevere in these environments. For instance, Jayla states the following, "I feel proud because, it's like Black and I'm proud, not just because people said it, like made it up or something, because it's true. So, as you think about it, if you go back to your ancestors and stuff, you have a big part of history. That's important, but like actually prove to people that we're not who you think we are, or like not just like judging because of the color of our skin. We're proud baby."

Zoe and others then state:

Zoe*:* Adding onto that, I feel like ever since like the 1800s till now, I think like the Black community has been like a huge empire, spreading over like the time back from slavery, you know, segregation, and now – and just like over time, like building up, coming more together. Hannah: It should also be more Black representation.

Tasha: In the book?

Nikia: The only time I've noticed that like over the years, most of the time, the only time you actually talk about Black history is Black history month, I don't think that's right. I mean, I understand Black history month, we're honoring like all the African Americans that died for us. We need to talk about that, like not just for one month.

Janae: Because they fought for our rights, and if they didn't fight for our rights, we would still be – half of us wouldn't even be here, because half of our ancestors would not have been either – would have been dead. And we would just have been – life would be horrible.

Hannah: Right, for us, yes.

Nikia: My name is Nikia. I am proud. Because it makes you feel like you can do anything, because you know that our African American ancestors did great things, so it makes you feel like, oh, I can do anything, because I am African American.

5.4.3 *Resilience: Still I Rise*

Despite Black girls' experiences within these school settings, Black girls emphasized the importance of space and sisterhood as they navigated racist and sexist school settings. For instance, Black girls discussed the importance of creating Black girl space and the importance of Black girl friendships to help them navigate White space. Black girl friendships are noted as necessary in predominately and racially and ethnically diverse schools.

Aaliyah: Well, most of my friends are Black, so sometimes our peers do treat most of us differently. When we're like around each other, just by ourselves, we can like act like ourselves. But some people might say we are ghetto, but like when we're like around other people, some of us have to act proper, because people might like call us ghetto or something. Akelee: Um, so it's a group of girls I hang with, they all Black and stuff, so like when it comes to us, we consider our friendship close.

Table 5.5 Themes, codes, and definitions

Codes	Definitions
Racial pride	Being proud to be black and being proud of the significant accomplishments of black Americans
Self-acceptance	Black girls are comfortable with who they are as a student of color within the school setting
Black girl friendships	Black girls enjoying forging friendships amongst themselves, where they are allowed to be and feel free
Black girl space	Intentionally creating black girl space where they can be themselves without judgment
Coping mechanism	Involves coping responses to behavior and actions of others within the school setting. More specifically, this may involve accepting offensive behavior and handling it by themselves and not informing authority figures. This can also involve ignoring offensive comments. Coping can involve confrontation and/or informing authority figures to not speaking out against it

Aaliyah: You can be yourself. Like you know that if you're doing something like. I don't know, you won't get judged for what you're doing. Because, like oh, these certain group of people do the same things as me, so it's like we are all the same.

Ke'era: My name is Ke'era. I am proud. Because it makes you feel like you can do anything, because you know that our African American ancestors did great things, so it makes you feel like, oh, I can do anything, because I am African American.

Summer: I look forward to seeing Black girls in higher every – in higher, um, in higher parts of the world, and, you know, getting all up to the, uh, big spots. Black girls having big businesses, because, you know, I look forward to putting myself in businesses, like having like my own lawyer department, big old building and stuff.

Collectively, while Black girls note the negative experiences within the classroom, they also talk about the importance of representation, creating Black girl space, and the importance of friendships and racial pride. In this instance, Black girls across the different educational spaces highlight what is needed and how they must continue envisioning a Black girl-centered future, as articulated by Summer (Table 5.5).

Overall, the findings corroborate previous literatures highlighting the significance of racial pride, friendships, and the necessity of creating space (Butler-Barnes et al., 2018; Kelly, 2018, 2020; Rogers & Butler-Barnes, 2021). The findings of this study highlight the significance of centering Black girls' voices to understand the way in which they cope with daily stressors due to racism and sexism and the importance of Black girl friendships. Thus, by continuing to center Black girls' voices could lead to anti-racist and anti-sexist to address their marginalization in the classroom.

5.5 Discussion

The current research aimed to explore the educational backgrounds of Black girls in a variety of educational institutions. We defined diversity as the presence of Black girls at schools with a majority White student body, a majority Black student body, and a student body that is comprised of students from a variety of other racial and ethnic backgrounds. The results showed that there were some commonalities across educational settings, such as the fact that Black females faced racist and sexist treatment in both predominantly White and racially and ethnically diverse settings. When compared to their non-Black counterparts, Black females discussed the negative stereotypes about them and treatment from their peers. These results are consistent with the research that shows that Black girls face unjust treatment in the classroom (Morris, 2007, Morris, 2016) and are subjected to harmful racial and sexist stereotypes, such as being called ghetto, loud, and stupid (Carter-Andrews et al., 2019; Morris, 2007). This study demonstrates these kinds of biases against Black girls are present in a variety of educational settings. Using the Integrative Model for the Developmental Competencies of Minority Children (García-Coll et al., 1996) as a guide, we may see the school setting as an environment that either fosters or stifles positive developmental competencies. These stories illustrate how schools may be hostile environments for Black girls, based on their social standing in terms of race and gender. However, by employing BFT, it was possible to put the experiences of Black girls in these contexts at the forefront, highlighting their efforts to resist, reclaim, and build Black girl space and friendships. Despite the difficulties they faced at school, Black girls stressed the value of racial pride, self-acceptance, companionship, and a safe place for Black girls to congregate. Below, we talk about the significance of these findings and why it is crucial to continue to elevate and provide space for the voices of Black females.

Our research confirms what others have written about the challenges Black girls face in the classroom. As has been widely noted, Black girls are disproportionately subject to punishment (Blake et al., 2011, 2022; Epstein et al., 2017). Teachers tend to have a negative impression of Black girls' intelligence (Gadson & Lewis, 2022; Ray, 2022). Black females are more likely to be suspended from school, both inside and outside of the classroom (Morris, 2016; Pelet del Toro, 2018; Wun, 2016).

Finally, research has revealed the racist and sexist stereotypes that Black females face on a daily basis (Annamma et al., 2019; Blake et al., 2011; Burnett et al., 2020; Morris, 2007; Townsend et al., 2010; Woodson, 2020). Because Black girls in this study reported being stereotyped as ghetto and dealing with racism and sexism, this research adds to the existing body of scholarship on this topic.

5.5.1 Black Girlhood: Resilience and Reclaiming

The results shed light on certain problematic aspects of the educational experiences of Black girls in a variety of contexts. Black girls shared strategies for thriving and succeeding in a variety of educational environments, each of which posed unique challenges to their identities and academic pursuits. A central topic was the importance of providing a safe space for Black girls in these communities. Black girls emphasized the need of creating safe spaces where they could be themselves and be supported by other Black girls. Black girls agreed that talking about Black history should not be confined to 1 month a year, but rather should be an integral part of the curriculum year-round.

These results support earlier research stressing the need for culturally relevant programming for Black girls. As an example, Gibbs Grey and Harrison (2020) discovered that Black girls who participated in a mentorship program were more likely to challenge unfair disciplinary practices at school and retell their own stories in their own voices, disputing the narratives that were told about them. Sister Nia is a culturally relevant program for African American girls that has been shown to have a positive effect on the participants' sense of self and identity (Belgrave et al., 2004). Toliver (2022) discovered that when Black girls participated in a writing workshop that emphasized narrating stories, they were better able to challenge negative and inconsistent self-perceptions. The perception of science among Black females was studied by Wade-Jaimes et al. (2021). They discovered that non-formal, after-school activities gave Black girls an opportunity to explore their own scientific identities and imagine themselves in the field outside of the traditional academic day.

Black girls' sisterhood and friendships were also crucial to thriving in these environments. This research implies that Black girl friendship is significant in settings where Black girls are in the minority, which is significant given the media's often unfavorable portrayal of relationships between Black girls. This is a significant finding given the common media portrayal of Black women and girls as antagonistic (Muhammad & McArthur, 2015). To date, there has not been any research on the benefits of Black girl friendships (Leath et al., 2022, but see Leath et al., 2021 and Leath et al., 2022 for exceptions). Leath et al. (2022) found that friendships with other Black women were identified as particularly meaningful by Black undergraduates in a study of students at a mostly White university. Having these friendships helped Black women feel more confident in who they were and less isolated as they dealt with bigotry and discrimination. Leath et al. (2021) conducted a study that looked backward at the friendship patterns of Black women throughout their time in high school. Friends of a different race were difficult to come by if those friends did not accept and validate their own racial and gender identities. Black women emphasized the value of racial pride and communal support. The importance of racial pride among Black girls has also been shown in studies. In a longitudinal study of Black girls, Butler-Barnes et al. (2018) found that racial pride was linked to greater intellectual interest.

The findings also revealed the value of Black girls organizing within their communities to combat injustice. For instance, one student emphasized the significance of having preachers visit the school and other members to help combat injustice. To combat racial disparities in public education, Jordan and Wilson (2017) highlight the positive effects when Black churches form school and church collaborations. Further research is warranted to learn about Black girls' social networks in schools and neighborhoods. These results have ramifications for other support institutions that can help reduce educational inequities, such as adult mentors and community activists. Last but not least, Black girls emphasized the significance of including Black history in the classroom. According to research by Scott et al. (2015), Black girls benefit from a culturally responsive computing program (COMPUGIRLS) because of the program's emphasis on the participants' actual experiences.

According to Ladson-Billings (2014), culturally responsive pedagogy is vital to the development of a positive self-image among Black youth. This requires maintaining a pedagogy that is culturally relevant and actively engages in equity and justice. Collectively, these results highlight the need for Black girl-specific educational environments, racial pride, Black girl friendships, and culturally sensitive teaching and content.

5.5.2 Limitations

The study's strength is the within-group analysis of Black girls from varying socioeconomic backgrounds who attended schools with racially and ethnically mixed student bodies. Yet, the research has some limitations. The student's race or ethnicity was not asked.

Similarly, to knowing the racial and ethnic makeup of one's classmates, knowing the racial and ethnic makeup of one's teachers would have supplied additional context. We also asked general questions on the school as a whole rather than specific questions regarding classroom experiences and the racial climate of the school. Moreover, when discussing their experiences, Black girls often generalized about the lives of all Black students, rather than identifying which Black students they were referring to. In addition, there was no information on how Black girls who identified as LGBTQI+ were treated in these institutions. Moving forward, it's crucial to understand the social identities of Black girls and the manifestations of the intersecting identities in mostly Black, predominantly White, or racially and ethnically diverse educational environments.

5.5.3 Implications for Understanding Family Resilience

The findings of this study show that Black girls' voices should be prioritized in school settings. It is equally critical that when Black girls are encountering difficulties at school, their parents be included within the school context. Furthermore, the scholarship has noted the types of racial socialization messaging that Black girls are receiving in order to cope with racialized stressors. For example, a plethora of research has found that racial socialization messages communicated to Black girls are associated with greater understanding about racial barriers and stressors that they must face in the environment (Butler-Barnes et al., 2018; Hughes et al., 2006; Stokes et al., 2020). There has also been a plethora of research that has documented how racial socialization functions as a protective mechanism for Black children who are exposed to racism at school (Dotterer et al., 2009; Saleem & Byrd, 2021; Wang & Huguley, 2012). These findings from this scholarship demonstrate the importance of "the talk" for Black girls, and as this work progresses, it is critical that Black parents understand what is going on within school settings, and that there be space where Black girls can engage in conversations that will lead to them having a healthier well-being.

5.5.4 Implications for Understanding Practice

The implications for practice include the importance of creating culturally responsive programming that supports the voice of Black girls and allows them to express themselves authentically. Rogers and Butler-Barnes (2022), for example, studied Black girls in a predominantly Black girl school context. The findings revealed that Black girls valued that space, that they recognized they could be their authentic selves, and that Black girls wanted additional programming where they could talk about some of the issues they were facing in the larger school setting.

Furthermore, the findings revealed that Black girls knew they could be themselves in that space. There has also been research conducted to demonstrate the significance of the creation of Black girl space (Belgrave et al., 2004; Inniss-Thompson et al., 2022). For example, Belgrave et al. (2004) created Sisters of Nia, a culturally relevant empowerment program aimed specifically at Black girls. Throughout the program, she noticed an increase in the Black girls' self-esteem, pride in their gender identities, and pride in their ethnic identities. As a result of these findings, it is clear how important it is for programming to be culturally appropriate. In addition to specific types of programming, organizations that serve young people and have populations of Black girls must listen to the girls' voices in order to identify the kind of programming that is most beneficial to them. To put it another way, this programming should be driven by young people, especially specifically Black girls.

5.5.5 Conclusion and Future Directions

In general, we add to the existing literature on the topic of Black girls' educational experiences. Black girls from a range of socioeconomic backgrounds and from districts with racially and ethnically diverse student populations made up our sample. We used Black Feminist Theory and the Integrative Model for the Developmental Competencies of Minority Children to put the voices of Black girls at the forefront of our work. As we move forward, it will be crucial to continue giving a platform to Black girls' voices and using theories that allow us to appreciate and comprehend their experiences. Further, Black girls should be seen as individuals rather than a collective, as they are the experts on their own lives and the best sources of information. The findings also have significance for interventions targeted on Black girls. For instance, Black girls emphasized the importance of friendships, racial pride, and the cultivation of a space dedicated to Black girlhood in their responses. In spite of having to contend with negative racist and gendered experiences within the classroom setting, it is possible that these factors should be investigated further as potential protective mechanisms for the purpose of building resiliency among Black girls. Further, the results of this research suggest that anti-blackness and anti-sexism should be at the core of professional development training for educators. Allowing Black girls to carve out their own niche in classrooms, especially in settings where they are the minority, is also crucial. This is a great chance to empower Black girls by providing them with a welcoming environment in which to share their perspectives and ideas. Being a Black girl is an integral component of identity, and the lessons learned in the classroom have a profound impact on how these young girls see themselves. Black girls can thrive in school if places are created that recognize their advantages while also addressing the obstacles they face.

Questions for Thought and Discussion

1. In thinking about centering Black girl voices to understand their lived experiences, what are some strategies that practitioners and educators do to ensure that Black girls voices are heard? What must practitioners and educators be aware of when working with Black girls?
2. Why is it important to understand the historical treatment of Black girls in the United States? What does this offer the practitioner and educator in working with Black girls?
3. Why it important to consider both race and gender when working with Black girls? What is the risk when practitioners or educators not considering the intersection of race and gender for Black girls?

Glossary of Terms

- *Intersectionality*: is confluence of race, gender, and class, are subjected to a multiplicity of kinds of oppression and marginalization.
- *Misogynoir*: The intersection of racism & sexism that produces racialized gendered violence.
- *Racism*: is the root cause of both prejudice and discrimination, which can be defined as the formation of unfavorable attitudes or beliefs regarding members of other racial groups and the discriminating treatment of members of these groups by both people and societal institutions.
- *Sexism*: Sexism is a form of prejudice or discrimination that is founded on misconceptions about a person's sex or gender.
- *STEM*: Science, Technology, Engineering, and Mathematics.

Conflict of Interest I have no known conflict of interest to disclose

References

Annamma, S. A., Anyon, Y., Joseph, N. M., Farrar, J., Greer, E., Downing, B., & Simmons, J. (2019). Black girls and school discipline: The complexities of being overrepresented and understudied. *Urban Education, 54*(2), 211–242.

Belgrave, F. Z., Reed, M. C., Plybon, L. E., Butler, D. S., Allison, K. W., & Davis, T. (2004). An evaluation of sisters of Nia: A cultural program for African American girls. *Journal of Black Psychology, 30*(3), 329–343. https://doi.org/10.1177/0095798404266063

Blake, J. J., Butler, B. R., Lewis, C. W., & Darensbourg, A. (2011). Unmasking the inequitable discipline experiences of urban black girls: Implications for urban educational stakeholders. *Urban Review, 43*(1), 90–106. https://doi.org/10.1007/s11256-009-0148

Blake, J. J., Jackson, L., Ruffin, N., Salter, P., Li, H., Banks, C., & Williams, K. S. (2022). Black girls and school discipline: The role of teacher's race, pubertal development, and discipline philosophy on discipline decisions. *Journal of Emotional and Behavioral Disorders, 30*(2), 128–137. https://doi.org/10.1177/10634266221077896

Burnett, M., Kurtz-Costes, B., Vuletich, H. A., & Rowley, S. J. (2020). The development of academic and nonacademic race stereotypes in African American adolescents. *Developmental Psychology, 56*(9), 1750–1759. https://doi.org/10.1037/dev0001071

Butler-Barnes, S. T., Leath, S., Williams, A., Byrd, C., Carter, R., & Chavous, T. M. (2018). Promoting resilience among African American girls: Racial identity as a protective factor. *Child Development, 89*(6), e552–e571. https://doi.org/10.1111/cdev.12995

Butler-Barnes, S. T., Lea, C. H., Leath, S., & Colin, R. (2019a). Voluntary interdistrict choice program: Examining black girls' experiences at a predominately white school. *Urban Review, 51*(2), 149–176. https://doi.org/10.1007/s11256-018-0464-y

Butler-Barnes, S. T., Richardson, B. L., Chavous, T. M., & Zhu, J. (2019b). The importance of racial socialization: School-based racial discrimination and racial identity among African American adolescent boys and girls. *Journal of Research on Adolescence, 29*(2), 432–448. https://doi.org/10.1111/jora.12383

Butler-Barnes, S. T., Lea, C. H., Leath, S., Rogers, L. O., Barnes, D. L., & Ibram, H. (2021). Visible or invisible? Black girls' experiences in a mathematics classroom. *Journal of African American Women and Girls in Education, 1*(2), 26–59. https://doi.org/10.21423/jaawge-v1i2a85

Butler-Barnes, S. T., Leath, S., Inniss-Thompson, M. N., Allen, P. C., D'Almeida, M. E. D. A., & Boyd, D. T. (2022). Racial and gender discrimination by teachers: Risks for black girls' depressive symptomatology and suicidal ideation. *Cultural Diversity and Ethnic Minority Psychology, 28*(4), 469–482. https://doi.org/10.1037/cdp0000538

Carter Andrews, D. J., Brown, T., Castro, E., & Id-Deen, E. (2019). The impossibility of being "perfect and white": Black girls' racialized and gendered schooling experiences. *American Educational Research Journal, 56*(6), 2531–2572. https://doi.org/10.3102/0002831219849392

Charmaz, K. (2002). Grounded theory analysis. In J. F. Gubrium & J. A. Holstein (Eds.), *Handbook of interview research* (pp. 675–694). Sage.

Chavous, T. M., Rivas-Drake, D., Smalls, C., Griffin, T., & Cogburn, C. (2008). Gender matters, too: The influences of school racial discrimination and racial identity on academic engagement outcomes among African American adolescents. *Developmental Psychology, 44*(3), 637–654. https://doi.org/10.1037/0012-1649.44.3.637

Coll, C. G., Crnic, K., Lamberty, G., Wasik, B. H., Jenkins, R., Garcia, H. V., & McAdoo, H. P. (1996). An integrative model for the study of developmental competencies in minority children. *Child Development, 67*(5), 1891–1914. https://doi.org/10.1111/j.1467-

Collins, P. H. (2000). *Black feminist thought*. Routledge.

Crenshaw, K. (1989). Demarginalizing the intersection of race and sex: A black feminist critique of antidiscrimination doctrine, feminist theory, and anti-racist politics. *University of Chicago Legal Forum, 1989*(1), 139–168.

Crenshaw, K. W. (1995). Mapping the margins: Intersectionality, identity politics, and violence against women of color. In K. Crenshaw, N. Gotanda, G. Peller, & K. Thomas (Eds.), *Critical race theory: The key writings that formed the movement* (pp. 357–383). The New Press.

Creswell, J. W. (2012). *Qualitative inquiry and research design: Choosing among five approaches*. Sage.

Dotterer, A. M., McHale, S. M., & Crouter, A. C. (2009). Sociocultural factors and school engagement among African American youth: The roles of racial discrimination, racial socialization, and ethnic identity. *Applied Development Science, 13*(2), 61–73. https://doi.org/10.1080/10888690902801442

Epstein, R., Blake, J. J., & González, T. (2017). *Girlhood interrupted: The erasure of Black girls' childhood.* Georgetown Law Center on Poverty and Inequality. https://www.blendedandblack.com/wp-content/uploads/2017/08/girlhood-interrupted.pdf

Esposito, J., & Edwards, E. B. (2018). When black girls fight: Interrogating, interrupting, and (re) imagining dangerous scripts of femininity in urban classrooms. *Education and Urban Society, 50*(1), 87–107. https://doi.org/10.1177/0013124517729206

Gadson, C. A., & Lewis, J. A. (2022). Devalued, overdisciplined, and stereotyped: An exploration of gendered racial microaggressions among black adolescent girls. *Journal of Counseling Psychology, 69*(1), 14–26. https://doi.org/10.1037/cou0000571

Gibbs Grey, T. M. D., & Harrison, L. M. (2020). Call me worthy: Utilizing storytelling to reclaim narratives about black middle school girls experiencing inequitable school discipline. *Equity and Excellence in Education*, 325–341. https://doi.org/10.1080/10665684.2020.1764880

Hughes, D., Rodriguez, J., Smith, E. P., Johnson, D. J., Stevenson, H. C., & Spicer, P. (2006). Parents' ethnic-racial socialization practices: A review of research and directions for future study. *Developmental Psychology, 42*(5), 747–770. https://doi.org/10.1037/0012-1649.42.5.747

Ibrahim, H., Barnes, D. L., Butler-Barnes, S. T., & Johnson, O., Jr. (2021). Impact of in-school suspension on black girls' math course-taking in high school. *Social Sciences, 10*, 272. https://doi.org/10.3390/socsci10070272

Inniss-Thompson, M., Butler-Barnes, S., Taaffe, C., & Elliott, T. (2022). "What serves you": Charting black girl spaces for wellness through spirituality, resistance, and homeplace. *Journal of African American Women and Girls in Education, 2*(2), 37–64.

Jordan, D. H., & Wilson, C. M. (2017). Supporting African American student success through prophetic activism: New possibilities for public school–church partnerships. *Urban Education, 52*(1), 91–119. https://doi.org/10.1177/0042085914566098

Kelly, L. L. (2018). A snapchat story: Now black girls develop strategies for critical resistance in school. *Learning, Media and Technology, 43*(4), 374–389. https://doi.org/10.1080/17439884.2018.1498352

Kelly, L. L. (2020). "I love us for real": Exploring homeplace as a site of healing and resistance for black girls in schools. *Equity & Excellence in Education, 53*(4), 449–464. https://doi.org/10.1080/10665684.2020.1791283

Ladson-Billings, G. (2014). Culturally relevant pedagogy 2.0: a.k.a. the remix. *Harvard Educational Review, 84*(1), 74.

Leath, S., Pfister, T., Ball, P., Butler-Barnes, S. T., & Evans, K. A. (2021). A qualitative exploration of school racial diversity, friendship choices, and black women's identity-based experiences in high school. *Journal of School Psychology, 89*(July 2020), 34–50. https://doi.org/10.1016/j.jsp.2021.09.006

Leath, S., Mims, L., Evans, K. A., Parker, T., & Billingsley, J. T. (2022). "I can be unapologetically who I am": A study of friendship among black undergraduate women at PWIs. *Emerging Adulthood, 10*(4), 837–851. https://doi.org/10.1177/21676968211066156

Mills, S. (2016). Caught between sexism, anti-sexism and `political correctness': Feminist women's negotiations with naming practices. *Discourse & Society, 14*(1), 87–110. https://doi.org/10.1177/0957926503014001931

Milner IV, H. R. (2007). Race, Culture, and Researcher Positionality: Working Through Dangers Seen, Unseen, and Unforeseen. *Educational Researcher*. https://doi.org/10.3102/0013189X07309471

Morris, E. W. (2007). "Ladies" or "ladies?": Perceptions and experiences of black girls in classrooms. *Youth and Society, 38*(4), 490–515. https://doi.org/10.1177/0044118X06296778

Morris, M. W. (2016). *Pushout: The criminalization of black girls in schools*. New Press.

Muhammad, G. E., & McArthur, S. A. (2015). "Styled by their perceptions": Black adolescent girls interpret representations of black females in popular culture. *Multicultural Perspectives, 17*(3), 133–140. https://doi.org/10.1080/15210960.2015.1048340

Nunn, M. N. (2018). Super-girl: Strength and sadness in black girlhood. *Gender and Education, 30*(2), 239–258. https://doi.org/10.1080/09540253.2016.1225013

Onyeka-Crawford, A., Patrick, K., & Chaudhry, N. (2017). *Let her learn: Stopping school pushout for girls of color.* National Women's Law Center. https://nwlc.org/resource/stopping-school-pushout-for-girls-of-color/

Pelet del Toro, V. M. (2018). Let black girls learn: Perceptions of black femininity and zero-tolerance policies in schools. *Revista Juridica de la Universidad de Puerto Rico, 87*, 55–74.

Ray, R. (2022). School as a hostile institution: How black and immigrant girls of color experience the classroom. *Gender and Society, 36*(1), 88–111. https://doi.org/10.1177/08912432211057916

Rogers, L. O., & Butler-Barnes, S. T. (2021). Black lives matter!: Systems of oppression affecting black youth: "[E]ven though we don't have everything…we build our own thing": Exploring black girl space. *Journal of Research on Adolescence, 2*(1), 49–68. https://doi.org/10.1111/jora.12697

Rogers, L. O., Butler Barnes, S., Sahaguian, L., Padilla, D., & Minor, I. (2021). # BlackGirlMagic: Using multiple data sources to learn about Black adolescent girls' identities, intersectionality, and media socialization. *Journal of Social Issues, 77*(4), 1282–1304. https://doi.org/10.1111/josi.12483

Saleem, F. T., & Byrd, C. M. (2021). Unpacking school ethnic-racial socialization: A new conceptual model. *Journal of Social Issues, 77*(4), 1106–1125. https://doi.org/10.1111/josi.12498

Scott, K. A., Sheridan, K. M., & Clark, K. (2015). Culturally responsive computing: A theory revisited. *Learning, Media and Technology, 40*(4), 412–436. https://doi.org/10.1080/17439884.2014.924966

Simmons, L. M. (2015). *Crescent City girls: The lives of young black women in segregated New Orleans*. University of North Carolina Press.

Smith-Evans, L., George, J., Graves, F. G., Kaufmann, L. S., & Frohlich, L. (2014). *Unlocking opportunity for African American girls: A call to action for educational equity.* National Women's Law Center. https://nwlc.org/wp-content/uploads/2015/08/unlocking_ opportunity_executive_summary.pdf

Stokes, M. N., Hope, E. C., Cryer-Coupet, Q. R., et al. (2020). Black girl blues: The roles of racial socialization, gendered racial socialization, and racial identity on depressive symptoms among black girls. *Journal of Youth and Adolescence, 49*, 2175–2189. https://doi.org/10.1007/s10964-020-01317-8

Strauss, A., & Corbin, J. (1998). *Basics of qualitative research techniques* (4th ed.). Sage.

Toliver, S. R. (2022). "Dreamland": Black girls saying and creating space through fantasy worlds. *Girlhood Studies, 15*(1), 17–33. https://doi.org/10.3167/ghs.2022.150103

Townsend, T. G., Thomas, A. J., Neilands, T. B., & Jackson, T. R. (2010). "I'm no Jezebel; I am young, gifted, and black": Identity, sexuality, and black girls. *Psychology of Women Quarterly, 34*(3), 273–285.

Wade-Jaimes, K., King, N. S., & Schwartz, R. (2021). "You could like science and not be a science person": Black girls' negotiation of space and identity in science. *Science Education, 105*(5), 855–879. https://doi.org/10.1002/sce.21664

Wang, M. T., & Huguley, J. P. (2012). Parental racial socialization as a moderator of the effects of racial discrimination on educational success among African American adolescents. *Child Development, 83*(5), 1716–1731. https://doi.org/10.1111/j.1467-8624.2012.01808.x

Williams, D. R., & Mohammed, S. A. (2009). Discrimination and racial disparities in health: Evidence and needed research. *Journal of Behavioal Medicine, 32*, 20–47. https://doi.org/10.1007/s10865-008-9185-0

Woodson, A. N. (2020). Don't let me be misunderstood: Psychological safety, black girls' speech, and black feminist perspectives on directness. *Journal of Educational Psychology, 112*(3), 567–578. https://doi.org/10.1037/edu0000458

Wright, N. S. (2016). *Black girlhood in the nineteenth century*. University of Illinois Press.

Wun, C. (2016). Unaccounted foundations: Black girls, anti-black racism, and punishment in schools. *Critical Sociology, 42*(4–5), 737–750. https://doi.org/10.1177/0896920514560444

Chapter 6
American Indian/Alaska Native Identities and the Indian Child Welfare Act of 1978 (ICWA) as Viewed Through Cultural Resilience Theory

Virginia Drywater-Whitekiller

For centuries prior to colonization, American Indians/Alaska Natives employed formal governance structures that supported tribal cultural traditions and life pathways to best meet the distinct needs of their tribal communities. A factor that is distinctive to American Indians/Alaska Natives, as compared to other minoritized groups, is the increasing number of federal laws and Supreme Court rulings that are specific to this population. The historical foundation for these regulatory processes reaches back to 100 years of treaty-making when the original inhabitants of the United States governed themselves as separate, sovereign tribal entities. However, in a short period of time, these treaties were broken by the newly formed colonist government and resulted in enforced practices designed to assimilate Native peoples into mainstream society (Hacker & Haines, 2005). In a rapidly evolving world, tribal nations were left to grapple with a dominant power's intent to eradicate their existence through cultural genocide.

Despite federal assimilation and acculturation policies, many American Indians/Alaska Natives continue to employ ethnic identification, collective identities, and cultural preservation while navigating contemporary mainstream society (Wexler, & Burke, 2011). This fluid movement is referred to as cultural resilience, a theory that stems from a strengths-based perspective and is defined as Native populations using their to overcome challenges that were not common to traditional Indigenous life (Strand & Peacock, 2003). Collective identity signifies one's sense of belonging to a particular group and is centered on cultural resilience (Polletta & Jasper, 2001). Without cultural identity, cultural traditions and values would cease to exist for the descendants of North America's first human inhabitants. American Indians/Alaska Native identities are subjected to mainstream political processes, often not

V. Drywater-Whitekiller (✉)
Department of Social Work, Northeastern State University, Tahlequah, OK, USA
e-mail: longvs@nsuok.edu

J. M. Koch et al. (eds.), *Identity as Resilience in Minoritized Communities*, Emerging Issues in Family and Individual Resilience,
https://doi.org/10.1007/978-3-031-38977-1_6

by choice, but by necessity. Consequently, American Indians/Alaska Natives and their allies were instrumental in spearheading political advocacy that led to the passage of the Indian Child Welfare Act (1978). In short, the purpose of this federal law is to establish guidelines designed to preserve culture and tribal ethnic identities for the youngest and most vulnerable; namely, American Indian/Alaska Native children removed from their homes by the public child welfare system. There is a stark contrast between traditional child rearing in American Indian/Alaska Native communities and child rearing in colonized child welfare institutions and Anglo families. Consequently, the dominant public system perpetually failed to consider or support the process of enculturation which is needed to support identity formation in collective group members (Whitekiller-Drywater, 2006).

6.1 Identity, Politics, and the Impact of Cultural Resilience

6.1.1 Ethnic Identity

Erikson (1968) postulated that developing a sense of personal identity, or sense of self, is a key part of the psychosocial adolescent stage of development and is influenced by ethnic identity (Markstrom, 2010). It is important to note that ethnic identity is different than race as the latter emphasizes supposedly biological characteristics that can lead to racism in American Indian/Alaska Native child welfare adoption (Elder, 2018) and public health services (Gartner et al., 2021). Ethnic identity determines what role, if any, tribal culture, and associated values will have in the lives of individuals. Ethnic identity for American Indians/Alaska Natives is multi-dimensional and complex. Put simply, American Indians/Alaska Natives are *different*. For example, identity can be: (1) influenced by tribal family which can include those who are not blood related, but considered like kin in the community; (2) dependent upon acculturation and forced assimilation into mainstream society; (3) collective group membership per tribal nation statuses; and (4) dictated by the federal recognition standards set forth by Congress due to centuries of policymaking by the federal government (Edmo et al., 2016; Legal Information Institute, n.d.). Put succinctly, "No other ethnic or cultural group is so heavily regulated" and while some policies were enacted to the benefit of American Indians and Alaska Natives, most were not (Pevar, 1992).

6.1.1.1 Indigenous Identity Politics

The United States government has had a vested interest in suppressing ethnic identity of the original inhabitants of this land what is now considered the United States of America. The motivations for this are as varied and complicated as is the contemporary ethnic identity of American Indians/Alaska Natives. Historical narratives have ranged from presumed benevolence directed toward saving the Indians through identity transformations that mirrored the individuality of mainstream culture (Gordon, 1964), to providing formal education and training (Szasz, 2005), and saving impoverished children from physical demise (Fuchs & Havighurst, 1972). It is important to note that prior to colonization, traditions, values, and cultural pathways supported the formation of Indigenous governments (Carter, 2011) and connection to the land was crucial in knowing who one was as an Indigenous person (Whitekiller-Drywater, 2017). The United States entered into multiple treaties with sovereign tribal governments. However, the surreptitious progression of colonial rule dismantled Indigenous governments, and extrapolated natural resources that were held sacred by American Indians/Alaska Natives to support developing economic infrastructures (Anderson, 2014). This dissolution was not by happenstance.

The progression of a dominant colonial rule accomplished the dismantlement of Indigenous governments (LeBeau, 2009). Even yet, these methods were slow to expedite assimilation as American Indian/Alaska Native families were reticent to change who they were since their Indigenous identities had served and sustained their culture well for centuries before the interference of colonization (Dozier, 1951; Stremlau, 2011). The cultural resilience left governmental, religious, and other mainstream institutions to get about the business of accelerating assimilation. This culminated in the removal of American Indian/Alaska Native children from their homes and tribal communities and indoctrinating them into "civilization" (Unger, 1977; Woolford et al., 2014). A calculated plan was devised to remove American Indian/Alaska Native children from their tribal roots and place them in boarding schools.

Hailed as an answer to the "Indian problem," boarding schools were designed for assimilation purposes. The primary justification used for these removals was physical and educational neglect of American Indian/Alaska Native children, both of which correlated with poverty and poor socioeconomic outcomes (Pember, 2016). In short, the outside destruction of traditional pathways, forced removals from homelands, and the associated traumas of abuse left little to no sustainable economic opportunities for the first Americans. Some Native families saw boarding schools and their offering of education and training as an avenue for their children to have an easier path as compared to the struggles of their ancestors. However, later government reporting concluded that the promises of education and training were misrepresented as many children were not students, but rather were exploited as menial laborers (Newland, 2022). In regard to the historical context of colonizing parenting practices, white mothers reported supporting racist ideas regarding how American Indian and Alaska Native mothers parented, further supporting non-voluntary home removals to boarding schools (Jacobs, 2008). Furthermore, works such as, "*If we get the girls, we get race,*" exposed how some boarding schools educated young Native girls and women to be mothers who raised assimilated children (Devens, 1992). Equally divisive was the Friends of the Indians, an 1880s eastern reformist movement whose outward propaganda purported they held the best interest of American Indians/Alaska Natives. Meanwhile, these "Friends" served as mechanisms to pass the Dawes Act, a federal law that led to the continued breakup of western communal lands and Native families who were removed from their eastern original homelands to what is now known as Oklahoma (Love, 1991). But the trauma did not end with land displacement resulting in the loss of connection to homelands, but also continued with child removals from homes, families, and communities.

Aptly referred to as the Indian child welfare crisis, the 1960s and 1970s involved additional child removals initiated by the public child welfare system and the Bureau of Indian Affairs, yet again resulting in the disenfranchisement of children from their families, communities, and culture (Jacobs, 2013). Even today, this population suffers disproportionality in child welfare out-of-home placements and exceeds other minoritized groups in the United States (Woods & Summers, 2016) and the numbers continue to increase. Although representing only 1% of the entire population of children in the United States, American Indian/Alaska Native children encompass 2.7% of those in foster care (National Indian Child Welfare Association, 2021). This type of soul wounding is not one that can be easily overlooked or overcome as generations continue to deal with the aftermath of boarding school experiences (Gameon & Skewes, 2020; Solomon, et al., 2022; Trafzer et al., 2010), forced relocations (Walters et al., 2010), and public child welfare out-of-home placements (Lucero & Bussey, 2012). However, American Indians/Alaska Natives have endured and when possible, continue to utilize cultural resilience by transmitting knowledge to future generations of what it means to be Indigenous peoples.

6.1.1.2 Cultural Resilience

Cultural resilience, also referred to as cultural buffers, protective behavioral strategies, or protective factors (e.g., ethnic identity, family support, spiritual beliefs, elder teaching) addresses diverse strengths that lead to well-being in American Indian/Alaska Natives (Whitekiller-Drywater, 2006, 2010). Ethnic identity supports cultural resilience in that we learn who we are through environmental social interactions referred to as enculturation (Phinney & Ong, 2007). Whitbeck (2006) found that it is through family and community social systems that enculturation occurs, a process that leads to affirmation, belonging, and a positive sense of identity. The importance of belonging is found in Erikson's (1968) classic work on identity matters. Furthermore, Maslow's hierarchy of needs was reportedly inspired by the Blackfeet Nation's concepts and teachings based upon his time spent with the Blackfeet Nation (Feigenbaum & Smith, 2020), demonstrated the essentialness of belonging prior to an individual's advancement to esteem and self-actualization (Tahir, 2021). Belongingness has also been viewed as protective factor that aids in higher peer acceptance and lowered loneliness in multicultural school-aged children (Baskin et al., 2010). As children enter adolescence, Erikson (1963) posited that the identity versus role confusion stage is commonplace during adolescence. He theorized that with successful passage through the stage, a sense of self and personal identity is established. This results in fidelity wherein the person accepts and commits to others, an attribute found in collective culture.

Without ethnic identity, there is no cultural resilience. Therefore, child removals away from their tribal families and communities continue to threaten cultural survival. The historical factors of American Indian/Alaska Native children being removed from their families and communities and placed in boarding schools continues to cause generational cultural disconnect and identity confusion (Winder, 2019). In non-Native out-of-home placements, cultural dissimilarity between foster or adopted children and their caregivers can result in negative psychosocial outcomes, such as discrimination (Casey Family Programs, 2007) and increase the likelihood of juvenile court involvement (Watt & Kim, 2019). Yet, Anderson and Linares (2012) found placements where foster parents and the children in care are culturally similar support positive ethnic identity in children.

6.1.1.3 Life Stressors and Resilience

In their extensive review of the literature, Soto et al. (2022) reported on American Indian/Alaska Native youth risk factors (i.e., life stressors, severe trauma, family history of alcohol use) that influence multiple substance (i.e., commercial tobacco, alcohol, opioid, stimulants) and behavioral (e.g., gambling) addictions. When historical trauma and poor socioeconomic factors were prevalent, resilience for the young participants was found to be impeded and they were therefore at increased risk for addictive behaviors. Henson et al. (2017) reported on nine protective factors that prevented substance abuse for young Native people. The factors noted were current and/or future aspirations, personal wellness, positive self-image, self-efficacy, non-familial connectedness, family connectedness, positive opportunities, positive social norms, and cultural connectedness. Relatedly, strong ethnic identity has been noted as a protective factor in reducing tobacco, alcohol, and marijuana use among American Indian/Alaska Native youth (Unger et al., 2020). And when compared to their white counterparts, the different values found in tribal identity, pride, the importance of extended family, and the influence of collective culture served to curtail the potential for substance abuse (Stanley et al., 2018).

Cultural resilience was also found as beneficial in lowering poor mental health factors. Mousseau et al. (2014) found that American Indian youth who exhibited high levels of community-driven traditional values, such as benevolence, presented with less depressive symptoms. These findings echoed the work of Smokowski et al. (2014), who discovered that ethnic identity in children and youth, particularly as found in American Indian/Alaska Native collective culture, reduced internalizing mental health problems (e.g., depression and anxiety). Likewise, employing protective factors (e.g., resilience and cultural continuity) in American Indian youth has been used as a framework for suicide prevention science (Allen et al., 2022). Additionally, the protective roles of culture through social connections of rural American Indian/Alaska Native youth were proposed to aid in social adjustment (Markstrom et al., 2016). Finally, social service programs that employed cultural identification and trauma-informed healing have resulted in positive outcomes for the young American Indian/Alaska Native participants (Brown et al., 2016; Friesen, et al., 2015; Jaycox et al. 2018; Kulis et al., 2017; Urbaeva et al. 2017).

In summary, studies indicate strong ethnic identities serve as positive social outcomes for Native peoples by providing protective buffers that are essential for raising healthy children. This is something that American Indians/Alaska Natives have known since time immemorial. For children involved in the public child welfare system, the prolonged separation from their Native families and communities leads to cultural disconnect depriving them of resiliency that offers lifetime support (Ullrich, 2020). The federal government's solution was "to kill the Indian" in the child to "save" them from their life pathways and civilize them (Churchill, 2004). However, what was needed was the lack of political interference that would permit tribal nations to determine what was best for their families and communities. Consequently, political maneuvering was needed to stop cultural genocide for vulnerable American Indian/Alaska Native children which formed the basis for the Indian Child Welfare Act (U.S. Department of the Interior, 2016).

6.1.2 The Indian Child Welfare Act

In 1978, the federal Indian Child Welfare Act (ICWA) was passed as means to sustain American Indian/Alaska Native children in their tribal culture and communities. Prior to the ICWA's passage reports indicated that 25–35% of all American Indian/Alaska Native children were placed outside of their families and communities (Hill, 2007). Although this law did not rectify the damage that was decades in the making, moving forward, it offered hope that future generations of children in the child welfare system would not suffer the same demise. The strategy was that when a child was brought to the attention of the public child welfare system, and home removal was inevitable, a ranking order would determine where the child would be placed; this strategy was also applied in adoption procedures. The first order was for the child to be placed with their extended family; next was placement with their tribal nation members, and finally placement would be with members of other tribal nations (National Indian Law Library, n.d.). Another prominent distinction for American Indian/Alaska Native children refers to the use of active efforts as compared to the commonly applied reasonable efforts utilized by state public child welfare in case management. In short, reasonable efforts refer to what would be considered a reasonable amount of effort on the caseworker's part to provide the parents with services that would aid in reunification of the child with their parent(s). However, active efforts require that the case (Edwards, 2019) worker must assist the parent or parents or Indian custodian through each step of the case plan by whatever means is necessary. After the passage of the law in 1978, the ICWA Final Rule expounded upon the definition of active efforts by providing 11 specific practice examples to guide public child welfare workers in managing American Indian/Alaska Native cases. Two of the 11 exemplars included offering and employing all available and culturally appropriate family preservation strategies and facilitating the use of remedial and rehabilitative services provided by the child's tribe (U.S. Department of the Interior, 2016).

In addition to the already determined placement preferences provided by ICWA, the Final Rule set the framework for child welfare workers that that every consideration is given to the prevailing social and conditions of the child's tribe while working toward the goal of reunification with their family (U.S. Department of the Interior, 2016). For instance, the child welfare worker must assist the family through the steps of each case, including assisting them in accessing and creating resources, if needed, that are based upon the facts of the case (Bureau of Indian Affairs, n.d.). If active efforts were employed and failed, this must be substantiated by the court prior to the termination of parental rights (U.S. Department of the Interior, 2016).

6.1.2.1 Disproportionality Continues

The idea behind ICWA was a noble one. Essentially, there should not be a time when American Indian/Alaska Native children are placed away from their families and tribal communities. Therefore, the sustainment of cultural continuity would ensue. Despite ICWA's intentions, past and current outcomes do not indicate a decrease in the number of children placed out of their homes and communities (Edwards & Rocha Beardall, 2021; Puzzanchera & Taylor, 2021). To exemplify, according to the National Indian Child Welfare Association (2021):

- American Indian/Alaska Native children are four times more likely to be removed by state child welfare systems than non-Native children even when their families have similar presenting problems.
- 13 states have significant overrepresentation of American Indian/Alaska Native children in state foster care systems at a rate 14 times higher than the general population.
- 56% of adopted American Indian/Alaska Native children are adopted outside their families and communities.

Data solidify the concern that generations of American Indian/Alaska Native children and their future generations are being denied the opportunity to develop and employ the cultural resilience that is essential to their well-being (Fletcher et al., 2009). There are various explanations as to why, in the face of a decades-old federal law, the likelihood of removal is imminent. One practice that can lead to outside placements is referred to as surveillance bias. This occurs when families are brought to the attention of public child welfare system for neglect (i.e., associated with poverty) and educational neglect (Berman, 2018). And once the family is on the system's radar, the likelihood is increased that future system involvement will follow. Edwards and Rocha Beardall (2021) reported that at least 50% of Native children under the age of 18 will be investigated. And for American Indian/Alaska Native children residing in Minnesota, Alaska, South Dakota, North Dakota, and Oklahoma, all states with large Indigenous populations, being investigated by child protection was a common part of growing up. When compared to historical forced boarding school attendance, due to neglect, it appears very little has changed.

6.1.2.2 Indian Child Welfare Act Supreme Court Challenges

Today, out of home placement issues are compounded with numerous United States Supreme Court cases that challenge ICWA's constitutionality. Some earlier cases ended positively. For instance, ICWA was supported in the case of *Mississippi Band of Choctaw Indians v. Holyfield* (1989) when the Supreme Court upheld tribal court jurisdiction regardless of where the child resided over the state court. Later, portions of ICWA suffered a significant loss when the Supreme Court ruled that the rights of an Indian father do not apply when the father is not the custodial parent of the Indian child (*Adoptive Couple v. Baby Girl,* 2013). A third case which awaits U.S. Supreme Court ruling is *Brackeen v. Haaland*, (formerly known as *Brackeen v. Bernhardt,* 2019. https://scholar.google.com/scholar_case?case=6317200377589723425&hl=en&as_sdt=6,44&as_vis=1).[1] The latter involves a non-American Indian/Alaska Native couple who adopted a Navajo Dine/Cherokee child. The adoptive parents' claim that ICWA violates the equal protection clause (viz., that the couple who wants to adopt is being subjected to racial discrimination because they are white) has again placed ICWA under the legal microscope.[2]

Finally, these cases have focused primarily on the birth parents and the extended family and have brought into question what the best interest of the American Indian/Alaska Native child is and who gets to determine this. A factor that has been negated is the child's voice in their family's matter. Integral to collective culture communication processes, the sum of the parts, in essence the individual voices of family, community members, and the child, equals the collective whole (Rudy & Grusec, 2006). Trivedi (2021) posited that the child should have the right to family integrity, "The right of a family to make private decisions about what is best for the family unit, free from unwarranted state intervention" (p. 268). Collective decision making as a historical Indigenous approach encircles the needs of the child and includes extended and like-kin family members. This approach contrasts with the colonized inclusion of family participation which is nuclear and more individualized in nature (Whitekiller-Drywater, 2013). The potential for the application of family integrity in ICWA court cases is one for consideration. This could be especially relevant when combined with family group decision-making which is inclusive of family and community members in developing the case plan on needs and support for family reunification.

[1] Native American Rights Fund (2022). Brackeen headed to the U.S. Supreme Court. Legal Review, 47(1), 1–4.

[2] The Brackeen's are represented pro bono by the law firm, Gibson Dun, who according to the Native American Rights Fund (NARF) have demonstrated interest in undermining tribal nations' mineral rights and sovereignty, via the exploitation of American Indian Alaska Indian children.

6.2 Implications

6.2.1 Implications for Understanding American Indian/Alaska Native Family Resilience

To understand American Indian/Alaska Native family resilience, one must acquire knowledge regarding the historical and contemporary lived experiences of this population. It is further important to grasp the underpinnings of tribal sovereignty as applied to the 574 federally recognized tribes in the United States (National Conference on State Legislators, 2020). These sovereign nations have been impacted by similar historical experiences and socioeconomic outcomes; however, they also have very distinct differences (e.g., language, culture, locations, traditions, belief systems, and values). Today, it is not uncommon for the family composition to entail varying degrees of assimilation and an amalgamation of tribal and cultural representation. Thus, it is imperative to be cognizant of biases that are based upon majority society perceptions as we should not compare and make judgment on what constitutes an American Indian/Alaska Native family.

In social work, it is declared that families are the experts of their own lives. It is critical to ask questions with genuine interest to gain insight as to how professionals can best advocate for and assist diverse populations. This should be relevant to practice, evidenced-based research, and policy implications. Furthermore, understanding American Indian/Alaska Native family resilience should not begin with a deficit-focused approach, but is initiated with the foundation of assessing and ascertaining family strengths. In doing so, we can uncover accompanying resiliencies that serve as buffers in adversity, even in the most vulnerable populations. To aptly understand American Indian/Alaska Native family resilience, we must practice walking in cultural humility and being open to what we do not know. And we must be diligent in searching for truths especially when utilizing outside resources that reference this population. Literature and associated materials must be properly vetted as for centuries American Indian/Alaska Native narratives and historical accounts have been relayed that lack the voices and the lived experiences of their subjects (National Child Welfare Workforce Institute, 2022).

Finally, American Indian/Alaska Natives families are resilient as this population continues to survive and increase in number (United States Census Bureau, 2021). This is despite colonialism, forced land relocations, dismantling of Indigenous governments, war, disease, boarding schools, and out-of-home/tribal community child placements. In short, surviving is very different than thriving. This population faces issues that are exacerbated by poverty (National Congress of American Indians, n.d.), poor health indicators, and lower life expectancies (Centers for Disease Control and Prevention, n.d.). All of this is system-related and cultural matters cannot be negated, especially regarding the implications for related policies and the influence that political undermining can have upon cultural resilience.

6.2.2 *Implications for Practice and Policy*

There is an antiquated view of ICWA as a law was designed to promote racial exception for American Indians/Alaska Natives, is conflicted and harmful to those it was created to protect. Yablon-Zug (2020) argues that this approach is problematic. She also notes that since ICWA's inception, contemporary federal child welfare policies for all children have become more modernized by reflecting best practices of family preservation and cultural connections. This supports the claim that ICWA is the "gold standard" that should be followed for all families (National Center for Juvenile Justice, 2019). When compared to other established child welfare policies that are now culturally inclusive with preference for family and kin, ICWA is more accurately depicted as American Indian/Alaska Native's right to equal protection (Yablon-Zug, 2020).

Sargent (2017) expounded upon American Indians/Alaska Natives being categorized as a race that was reinforced by government census rolls that required the documentation of blood quantum. She posited that this was supported by the myth of Manifest Destiny which touted the superiority of colonists over the original inhabitants. Predictions were that with the mixing of other races, American Indians would thin their Native "blood" which would lead to a vanished race; race-making concerning American Indian/Alaska Native children continues to play out in state court systems (Brown, 2020). However, the expectation that American Indians/Alaska Natives would disappear has fallen short as this populace has experienced a population resurgence especially in the past decades (Shoemaker, 1999). Yet, forced assimilation continues in the vein of out-of-home placements and child adoptions that occur away from tribal family and communities. American Indian/Alaska Native nations continue to battle the hegemony of policies and court rulings that perpetually threaten their survival as a collective group of people. One implication for policy reformation was described by Beardall and Edwards (2021) who suggested American Indian/Alaska Native children be removed from the public child welfare system. Their alternative is simple one: allocate adequate resources to the tribal nations who can provide for the needs of the children and families. This is a prevention and intervention approach. In this way, tribes can truly exercise their sovereignty and self-determination while protecting the best interests of their children with cultural continuity based upon resilient practices, positive ethnic identities, and well-being.

6.3 Conclusion and Future Directions

As collective groups who share assumptions, values, and norms, American Indians/Alaska Natives have long battled the right to maintain their specific ethnic identities, a known supportive factor in family and cultural resilience. This struggle has been evident since the onset of colonization and has continued to gain momentum through challenges associated with the constitutionality of the Indian Child Welfare Act of 1978. Due to the association of poverty and related economic social outcomes, American Indian/Alaska Native children are at-risk for placement away from their homes, families, and tribal communities. For many, this will result in legal adoption into non-Native families and bears the strong likelihood that they will be reared in non-tribal communities, diminishing the opportunity for their generation and their future generations to know who they are as Indigenous peoples.

American Indians/Alaska Natives have withstood overt and covert political agendas designed to take from them what is most sacred, namely, their families, children, culture, and their lands. This should not be the case as treaty-making with the federal government recognized tribes as sovereign nations who had the authority to enter into nation-to-nation agreements with the United States. As the saying goes, treaties do not expire. Today, tribal members maintain citizenship with their federally recognized tribes, the United States, and the states in which they reside. While awaiting the outcome of the *Brackeen v. Haaland* case, an alarm is sounded throughout Indian Country as tribal nations and their allies are preparing to defend yet another assimilation attack.

When considering future directions, it is important to note that some tribal nations do administer their own child welfare agencies since the passage of ICWA in 1978. However, these organizations are poorly funded and cannot provide the holistic services needed to aptly care for all their families and children who are involved in the public child welfare system. To increase funding, there are a small number of tribes that have gone through the lengthy process of being approved for direct Title IV-E foster care. In short, Title IV-E is federal funding that is available to all the states whereas reimbursement can be received for a portion of foster care expenditures (Children's Bureau, n.d.). Still, there remains a need for current and future Title IV-E tribes to be granted the opportunity to use culturally inclusive interventions that will work in their communities. Additionally, when a child's custody is transferred from the state to the tribe, the funding that the state was receiving for the child should follow them to their Indian child welfare agency. Finally, assimilation of American Indian/Alaska Native peoples, the federal government's solution to the Indian "problem" did not involve those who are most impacted and had the most to gain or lose. The Indian Child Welfare Act was passed to reverse this type of blatant discrimination and must be upheld.

Questions for Thought and Discussion

1. In what ways can the IWCA serve as a model for maintaining family preservation, cultural connections, and improved child welfare in other minoritized communities?
2. In what ways do the enculturation of American Indian and Alaska Native youth serve to uphold the integrity and viability of their tribal nations?
3. Disregarded treaties have created a legacy of ongoing harm to American Indian and Alaska Native communities. What strategies for repair would be most effective?

4. What can service providers do to educate themselves in learning about and supporting the diverse cultural repertoires of the American Indian and Alaska Native citizens they serve/citizens with whom they interact?

Conflict of Interest I have no known conflict of interest to disclose

References

Adoptive Couple v. Baby Girl, 570 U.S. 637. (2013). https://supreme.justia.com/cases/federal/us/570/637/

Allen, J., Wexler, L., & Rasmus, S. (2022). Protective factors as a unifying framework for strength-based intervention and culturally responsive American Indian and Alaska Native suicide prevention. *Prevention Science: The Official Journal of the Society for Prevention Research, 23*(1), 59–72. https://doi.org/10.1007/s11121-021-01265-0

Anderson, G. C. (2014). *Ethnic cleansing and the Indian: The crime that should haunt America.* University of Oklahoma Press.

Anderson, M., & Linares, L. O. (2012). The role of cultural dissimilarity factors on child adjustment following foster placement. *Child Youth Services Review, 34*(4), 597–601. https://doi.org/10.1016/j.childyouth.2011.11.016

Baskin, T. W., Wampold, B. E., Quintana, S. M., & Enright, R. D. (2010). Belongingness as a protective factor against loneliness and potential depression in a multicultural middle school. *The Counseling Psychologist, 38*(5), 626–651. https://doi.org/10.1177/0011000009358459

Beardall, T. R., & Edwards, F. (2021). Abolition, settler colonialism, and the persistent threat of Indian child welfare. *Columbia Journal of Race and Law, 11*(3), 533–574. https://doi.org/10.52214/cjrl.v11i3.8744

Berman, M. (2018). Resource rents, universal basic income, and poverty among Alaska's Indigenous peoples. *World Development, 106*, 161–172.

Brackeen v. Bernhardt, 937 F.3d 406, 420 (5th Cir. 2019).

Brown, H. E. (2020). Who is an Indian child? Institutional context, tribal sovereignty, and race-making in fragmented states. *American Sociological Review, 85*(5), 776–805. https://doi.org/10.1177/0003122420944165

Brown, R. A., Dickerson, D. L., & D'Amico, E. J. (2016). Cultural identity among urban American Indian/Alaska Native youth: Implications for alcohol and drug use. *Prevention Science, 17*(7), 852–861. https://doi.org/10.1007/s11121-016-0680-1

Bureau of Indian Affairs. (n.d.). *Active efforts reference sheet.* https://tribalinformationexchange.org/files/products/ActiveEffortsResourceList.pdf

Carter, N. C. (2011). U.S. Federal Indian policy: An essay and annotated bibliography. *Legal Reference Services Quarterly, 30*, 210–230.

Casey Family Programs. (2007). *Mental health, ethnicity, sexuality, and spirituality among youth in foster care: Findings from the mental health Casey field study.* https://www.casey.org/media/MentalHealthEthnicitySexuality_FR.pdf

Centers for Disease Control and Prevention. (n.d.). *Health of American Indian or Alaska Native population.* FastStats – Health of American Indian or Alaska Native Population (cdc.gov)

Children's Bureau. (n.d.). *Title IV-E foster care eligibility reviews fact sheet.* Administration for Children and Families, U.S. Department of Health and Human Services. Title IV-E Foster Care Eligibility Reviews Fact Sheet | The Administration for Children and Families (hhs.gov)

Churchill, W. (2004). *Kill the Indian, save the man: The genocidal impact of American Indian residential schools.* City Lights.

Devens, C. (1992). "If we get the girls, we get the race": Missionary education of Native American girls. *Journal of World History, 3*(2), 219–237.

Dozier, E. P. (1951). Resistance to acculturation and assimilation in an Indian pueblo. *American Anthropologist, 53*(1), 56–66.

Edmo, S., Young, J., & Parker, A., (2016). American Indian identity: Citizenship, membership, and blood. In B. E. Johnson (Series Ed.), *Native American: Yesterday and today*. ABC-CLIO.

Edwards, L. (2019). Defining active efforts in the Indian Child Welfare Act. *The Guardian, 41*(1), 1–8.

Edwards, F., & Rocha Beardall, T. (2021, April 1). *American Indian and Alaska Native child welfare system contact across U.S. States: Magnitudes and mechanisms*. https://doi.org/10.31235/osf.io/fcz5p.

Elder, A. K. (2018). "Indian" as a political classification: Reading the tribe back into the Indian Child Welfare Act. *Northwestern Journal of Law & Social Policy, 13*(4), 417–438.

Erikson, E. H. (1963). *Youth: Change and challenge*. Basic books.

Erikson, E. H. (1968). *Identity: Youth and crisis*. W. W. Norton.

Feigenbaum, K. D., & Smith, R. A. (2020). Historical narratives: Abraham Maslow and Blackfoot interpretations. *Humanistic Psychologist, 48*(3), 232–243.

Fletcher, M. L., Singel, W. T., & Fort, K. E. (2009). *Facing the future: The Indian Child Welfare Act at flec30*. Michigan State University Press.

Friesen, B. J., Cross, T. L., Jivanjee, P., Thirstrup, A., Bandurraga, A., Gowen, L. K., & Rountree, J. (2015). Meeting the transition needs of urban American Indian/Alaska Native youth through culturally based services. *The Journal of Behavioral Health Services & Research, 42*(2), 191–205. https://doi.org/10.1007/s11414-014-9447-2

Fuchs, E., & Havighurst, R. J. (1972). *To live on this earth: American Indian education*. University of Albuquerque. New Mexico Press.

Gameon, J. A., & Skewes, M. C. (2020). A systematic review of trauma interventions in Native communities. *American Journal of Community Psychology, 65*(1–2), 223–241. https://doi.org/10.1002/ajcp.12396

Gartner, D. R., Wilbur, R. E., & McCoy, M. L. (2021). "American Indian" as a racial category in public health: Implications for communities and practice. *American Journal of Public Health, 111*(11), 1969–1975. https://doi.org/10.2105/AJPH.2021.306465

Gordon, M. M. (1964). *Assimilation in American life: The role of race, religion, and national origins*. Oxford University Press.

Hacker, J. D., & Haines, M. R. (2005). American Indian mortality in the late nineteenth century: The impact of federal assimilation policies on a vulnerable population. *Annals of Historical Demography, 110*(2), 17–29. https://doi.org/10.3917/adh.110.0017

Henson, M., Sabo, S., Trujillo, A., & Teufel-Shone, N. (2017). Identifying protective factors to promote health in American Indian and Alaska native adolescents: A literature review. *Journal of Primary Prevention, 38*, 5–26. https://doi.org/10.1007/s10935-016-0455-2

Hill, R. B. (2007). *An analysis of racial/ethnic disproportionality and disparity at the national, state, and county levels*. Casey-CSSP Alliance for Racial Equity in Child Welfare.

Indian Child Welfare Act of 1978, Pub.L. 95–608, 92 Stat. 3069, 25 U.S.C. §§ 1901–1963 (1978). https://www.govtrack.us/congress/bills/95/s1214

Jacobs, M. D. (2008). The great white mother: Maternalism and American Indian child removal in the American West, 1880–1940. In E. Jameson & S. McManus (Eds.), *One step over the line: Toward a history of women in the North American West* (pp. 190–213). University of Alberta Press.

Jacobs, M. D. (2013). Remembering the "forgotten child": The American Indian child welfare crisis of the 1960s and 1970s. *American Indian Quarterly, 37*(1–2), 136–159.

Jaycox, L., Langley, A., Hoover, S. A., & Jaycox, L. (2018). *Cognitive behavioral intervention for trauma in schools (CBITS) for American Indian youth* (2nd ed.). RAND Corporation.

Kulis, S. S., Ayers, S. L., & Harthun, M. L. (2017). Substance use prevention for urban American Indian youth: A efficacy trial of the culturally adapted living in 2 worlds program. *The Journal of Primary Prevention, 38*(1–2), 137–158. https://doi.org/10.1007/s10935-016-0461-4

LeBeau, P. R. (2009). *Term paper resource guide to American Indian history*. Greenwood Press.

Legal Information Institute. (n.d.). 25 CFR § 83.11 – *What are the criteria for acknowledgment as a federally recognized Indian tribe*? Cornell Law School. https://www.law.cornell.edu/cfr/text/25/83.11

Love, C. J. (1991). *The Friends of the Indians and Their Foes: A Reassessment of the Dawes Act Debate*. (*Honors Papers* No. 571). Oberlin College. https://digitalcommons.oberlin.edu/honors/571

Lucero, N. M., & Bussey, M. (2012). A collaborative and trauma-informed practice model for urban Indian child welfare. *Child Welfare, 91*(3), 89–112.

Markstrom, C. A. (2010). Identity formation of American Indian adolescents: Local, national, and global considerations. *Journal of Research on Adolescents, 21*(2), 519–535. https://doi.org/10.1111/j.1532-7795.2010.00690.x

Markstrom, C. A., Moilanen, K. L., & Crockett, L. J. (2016). Rural ethnic minority youth and families in the United States: Theory, research, and applications. In L. Crockett & G. Carlo (Eds.), *School, community, and cultural connectedness as predictors of adjustment among rural American Indian/Alaska Native (AI/AN) adolescents* (pp. 109–126). Springer International. https://doi.org/10.1007/978-3-319-20976-0_7

Mississippi Band of Choctaw Indians v. Holyfield, 109 S. Ct. 1597; 104 L. (Ed. 2d 29; 1989).

Mousseau, A. C., Scott, W. D., & Estes, D. (2014). Values and depressive symptoms in merican Indian youth of the northern plains: Examining the potential moderating roles of outcome expectancies and perceived community values. *Journal of Youth and Adolescence: A Multidisciplinary Research Publication, 43*(3), 426–436. https://doi.org/10.1007/s10964-013-9982-9

National Center for Juvenile Justice. (2019). *Disproportionality rates for children of color in foster care dashboard*. National Center for Juvenile Justice.

National Child Welfare Workforce Institute. (2022). *American Indian Alaska Natives curriculum content evaluation guide*. American Indian/Alaska Natives Curriculum Content Evaluation Guide – National Child Welfare Workforce Institute. ncwwi.org.

National Conference on State Legislators. (2020). *Federal and state recognized tribes*. List of Federal and State Recognized Tribes. ncsl.org

National Congress of American Indians. (n.d.). *Demographics: Indian country demographics*. Demographics | NCAI

National Indian Child Welfare Association. (2021). *Disproportionality in child welfare fact sheet*. National Indian Child Welfare Association. https://www.nicwa.org/wp-content/uploads/2021/12/NICWA_11_2021-Disproportionality-Fact-Sheet.pdf

National Indian Law Library. (n.d.). *ICWA guide online: Topic 16 placement*. http://www.narf.org/nill/documents/icwa/faq/placement.html

Newland, B. (2022). *Federal Indian boarding school initiative investigative report*. United States Department of the interior, Office of the Secretary. https://www.bia.gov/sites/default/files/dup/inlinefiles/bsi_investigative_report_may_2022_508.pd f

Pember, M. A. (2016). *Intergenerational trauma: Understanding Natives' inherited pain*. Indian Country Today Media Network.

Pevar, S. L. (1992). *The rights of Indians and tribes: The basic ACLU guide to Indian and tribal rights* (2nd ed.). Southern Illinois University Press.

Phinney, J. S., & Ong, A. D. (2007). Conceptualization and measurement of ethnic identity: Current status and future directions. *Journal of Counseling Psychology, 54*(3), 271–281.

Polletta, F., & Jasper, J. M. (2001). Collective identity and social movements. *Annual Review of Sociology, 27*(1), 283–305.

Puzzanchera, C., & Taylor, M. (2021). *Disproportionality rates for children of color in foster care* [Dashboard]. National Council of Juvenile and Family Court Judges. https://www.ncjj.org/AFCARS/Disproportionality_Dashboard.aspx

Rudy, D., & Grusec, J. (2006). Authoritarian parenting in individualist and collectivist groups: Associations with maternal emotion and cognition and children's self-esteem. *Journal of Family Psychology, 20*(1), 68–78. https://doi.org/10.1037/0893-3200.20.1.68

Sargent, S. (2017). Truth and consequences: Law, myth and metaphor in American Indian contested adoption. *Liverpool Law Review: A Journal of Contemporary Legal and Social Policy Issues, 38*(1), 47–61. https://doi.org/10.1007/s10991-017-9193-7/

Shoemaker, N. (1999). *American Indian population recovery in the twentieth century*. University of New Mexico Press.

Smokowski, P. R., Evans, C. B. R., Cotter, K. L., & Webber, K. C. (2014). Ethnic identity and mental health in American Indian youth: Examining mediation pathways through self-esteem, and future optimism. *Journal of Youth and Adolescence: A Multidisciplinary Research Publication, 43*(3), 343–355. https://doi.org/10.1007/s10964-013-9992-7

Solomon, T. G. A., Starks, R. R. B., Attakai, A., Molina, F., Cordova-Marks, F., Kahn-John, M., Antone, C. L., Flores, M., & Garcia, F. (2022). The generational impact of racism on health: Voices from American Indian communities. *Health Affairs (Project Hope), 41*(2), 281–288. https://doi.org/10.1377/hlthaff.2021.01419

Soto, C., West, A. E., Ramos, G. G., & Unger, J. B. (2022). Substance and behavioral addictions among American Indian and Alaska Native populations. *International Journal of Environmental Research and Public Health, 19*, 1–15. https://doi.org/10.3390/ijerph19052974

Stanley, L. R., Kelly, K. J., Swaim, R. C., & Jackman, D. (2018). Cultural adaptation of the be under your own influence media campaign for middle-school American Indian youth. *Journal of Health Communication, 23*(12), 1017–1025. https://doi.org/10.1080/10810730.2018.1536730

Strand, J. A., & Peacock, R. (2003). Resource guide: Cultural resilience. *Tribal College Journal, 14*(4), 28–31.

Stremlau, R. (2011). *Sustaining the Cherokee family: Kinship and the allotment of an indigenous nation*. University of North Carolina Press.

Szasz, M. C. (2005). "I knew how to be moderate and I knew how to obey": The commonality of American Indian boarding school experiences, 1750s–1920s. *American Indian Culture and Research Journal, 29*(4), 75–94.

Tahir, H. (2021). Exploration of self-actualization and belongingness in divergent through the lens of Maslow's hierarchy of needs. *Research Journal of Language and Literature, 6*(1), 1–24.

Trafzer, C. E., Keller, J. A., Sisquoc, L., & (Eds.). (2010). *Boarding school blues: Revisiting American Indian educational experiences*. University of Nebraska Press.

Trivedi, S. (2021). My family belong to me: A child's constitutional right to family integrity. *Harvard Civil Rights-Civil Liberties Law Review, 56*(2), 267–313.

U.S. Department of the Interior. (2016). *The ICWA final rule*. https://www.federalregister.gov/documents/2016/06/14/2016-13686/indian-child-welfare-act-proceedings

Ullrich, J. S. (2020). *Indigenous connectedness as a framework for relational healing within Alaska Native Child Welfare* (Doctoral dissertation). https://digital.lib.washington.edu/researchworks/handle/1773/45544

Unger, S. (1977). *The destruction of American Indian families*. Association on American Indian Affairs.

Unger, J. B., Sussman, S., Begay, C., Moerner, L., & Soto, C. (2020). Spirituality, ethnic identity, and substance use among American Indian/Alaska Native adolescents in California. *Substance Use & Misuse, 55*(7), 1194–1198. https://doi.org/10.1080/10826084.2020.1720248

United States Census Bureau. (2021). *Improved race and ethnicity measures reveal U.S. population is much more multiracial: 2020 Census illuminates racial and ethnic composition of the country*. United States Census Bureau. https://www.census.gov/library/stories/2021/08/improved-race-ethnicity-measures-reveal-united-states-population-much-more-multiracial.html

Urbaeva, Z., Booth, J. M., & Wei, K. (2017). The relationship between cultural identification, family socialization and adolescent alcohol use among Native American families. *Journal of Child and Family Studies, 26*(10), 2681–2693. https://doi.org/10.1007/s10826-017-0789-2

Walters, K. L., Beltran, R., Huh, D., & Campbell, T. E. (2010). Displacement and dis-ease: Land, place, and health among American Indians Alaska Natives. In L. M. Burton, S. Kemp, M. Leung, & S. A. Mathews (Eds.), *Communities, neighborhoods, and health: Social disparities in health and health care* (pp. 163–199). Springer. https://doi.org/10.1007/978-1-4419-7482-2_10

Watt, T., & Kim, S. (2019). Race/ethnicity and foster youth outcomes: An examination of disproportionality using the national youth in transition database. *Children and Youth Services Review, 102*, 251–258.

Wexler, L., & Burke, T. K. (2011). Cultural identity, multicultural competence and resilience: A pilot study of Alaska Native students' experience at university. *Journal of American Indian Education, 50*(2), 44–64.

Whitbeck, L. B. (2006). Some guiding assumptions and a theoretical model for developing culturally specific preventions with Native American people. *Journal of Community Psychology, 24*, 183–192.

Whitekiller-Drywater, V. (Fall, 2006). What this dominant society can't always give me: Perceptions of Native American elders teaching Native traditions. *Journal of Baccalaureate Social Work, 12*(1), 71–86.

Whitekiller-Drywater, V. (2010). Cultural resilience: Voices of native American students in college retention. *The Canadian Journal of Native Studies, 30*(1), 1–19.

Whitekiller-Drywater, V. (2013). Family group conferencing: An Indigenous practice approach to compliance with the Indian Child Welfare Act. *Journal of Public Child Welfare, 8*(3), 260–278. https://doi.org/10.1080/15548732.2014.907102

Whitekiller-Drywater, V. (2017). We belong to the land: Native Americans experiencing and coping with microaggressions. *The Canadian Journal of Native Studies, 37*(1), 153–174.

Winder, N. N. (2019). Colliding heartwork: The space where our hearts meet and collide to process the boarding school experience. In *Residential schools and indigenous peoples* (pp. 141–162). Routledge.

Woods, S., & Summers, A. (2016). *Technical assistance bulletin: Disproportionality rates for children of color in foster care* (Fiscal Year 2014). National Council of Juvenile and Family Court Judges.

Woolford, A. J., Benvenuto, J., & Hinton, A. L. (2014). *Colonial genocide in indigenous North America*. Duke University Press. https://doi.org/10.1215/9780822376149

Yablon-Zug, M. (2020). ICWA's irony. *American Indian Law Review, 45*(1), 1–88.

Chapter 7
African American Home/Schooling: Continuing a Legacy of Family and Educational Resilience

Stacie L. Warner

Historically, education has presented consistent challenges to Black, Indigenous, and People of Color (BIPOC). Academic scholarship highlights and magnifies the marginalization and disparity that children of color, especially Black children, have experienced in many schools across America since their development in the colonial era. Throughout the twentieth century, a significant portion of scholarship and research on educational inequities focused on the implications of educational marginalization, criminalization, and racism on Black boys (Ferguson, 2020); however, in recent years, scholarship has increasingly turned toward the educational relegation and criminalization of Black girls. The contributions of contemporary scholars like Kimberle' Crenshaw, Monique Morris, and Ruth Nicole Brown make it clear that Black girls are routinely disbarred from ideas of childhood, girlhood, and equitable education. As a result, public and private schools have become inequitable, problematic spaces for Black girls, much like their male counterparts. As a result of such realities for Black children, more Black families are opting to home/school to resist the disenfranchisement of Black students.

Homeschooling—referred to in varying ways such as home/schooling, home-based education, home education, home-centered learning, home instruction, deschooling, and unschooling—is generally linked to the idea of parents rejecting mainstream schooling and deciding to educate their children in a home or alternative setting (Murphy, 2012). Initially a necessity for the family and societal state, families have used the home to educate children since the beginning of American history (Williams, 2009). Different motivations have driven the choice to homeschool for different demographics of people. For millennia, Native Americans used homeschooling to educate the next generation of knowledge of the land and tribal

S. L. Warner (✉)
Oklahoma State University, Stillwater, OK, USA
e-mail: stacie.warner@okstate.edu

J. M. Koch et al. (eds.), *Identity as Resilience in Minoritized Communities*, Emerging Issues in Family and Individual Resilience,
https://doi.org/10.1007/978-3-031-38977-1_7

traditions (Lawrence, 2019). Largely driven by faith and few available schools, early settlers used home education for the first 40 years of the colony's existence (Gaither, 2017; Urban et al., 2019). For African American families, home/schooling continues a legacy of autonomy and liberatory practices that African Americans have embraced since slavery.

Utilizing Luther et al.'s (2000) definition of resilience as "a dynamic process encompassing positive adaptations within the context of significant adversity" (p. 543), this chapter explores how African American home/schooling continues a historical legacy of resilience salient to the efforts of Black people and parents to achieve educational freedom and distinction. This chapter posits that home/schooling fosters family resilience by allowing Black parents to enact counter-practices to the normative practices, ideals, and structures instituted by formal education while taking ownership of their children's education in a space that offers educational freedoms and possibilities. For the purpose of this chapter, family resilience is defined as the capacity of a family to overcome and withstand adversity, becoming stronger and more resourceful (Walsh, 2016). Additionally, the author will use the terms African American and Black interchangeably.

7.1 Homeschooling Scholarship

7.1.1 History of Homeschooling

Education stretches beyond teaching and learning. As anthropologist Tim Ingold (2018) posits, education is "whenever and wherever life is going on" (p. 3). The home serves as a site for some of a child's most meaningful education: survival, emotions/feelings, negotiation, gain, loss, morality, and self-care. Parents and guardians take on the tasks of Ingold's vision of a teacher: one who does not "…explicate knowledge for the benefit of those who are assumed, by default, to be ignorant, but to provide inspiration, guidance, and criticism in the exemplary pursuit of truth" (Ingold, 2017, n.p.). It is generally in the home where children learn as they live or "become" (Ingold, 2018). There has not been a time throughout American history when the home was not a foundational structure of children's education. Since its origins, there has been an evolution in homeschooling well documented throughout scholarship. Cremin (1970) presented some of the earliest historical scholarship on the phenomenon and identified the role of the home as a site for "sustained and systematic instruction" (p. 128).

Since Cremin's influential early publication, scholars have continued to expand their understanding of homeschooling's varied expressions and facets. Lois (2013) examines the lived experiences of mothers that choose to homeschool, and the role mothering plays in the practice. The findings of Lois' 10-year ethnographic study illuminate the often misunderstood and complex nature of homeschooling mothers, their motivations, and the social-psychological impact homeschooling has on the mothers. Detailing a history of homeschooling that spans the colonial period to the present, Gaither (2017) provides a comprehensive account of how people have used the home as a space for education of all kinds. Gaither highlights how homeschooling has and continues to evolve in its purposes, practices, and perceptions over time.

Greenwalt (2019) challenged readers to rethink homeschooling as something all families engage in and that public schools should embrace and support. Greenwalt (2019) posits that it is an illusion to think there is only one place to learn with one type of teacher; the home and the classroom are both essential sites of learning, and parents and teachers share a dual role in teaching and rearing. Expanding on historical homeschooling research, Dwyer and Peters (2019) discuss some philosophical, historical, and social beliefs surrounding home education and its positionality in twenty-first-century education. The authors provide an in-depth analysis of the varying beliefs and competing arguments surrounding the practice and offer the advocation of practices and policies that address the different sides of the homeschooling debate. As more families, parents, and guardians opt to homeschool for varying reasons, new scholarship continues to emerge on the phenomena.

Since roughly 2012, attention has focused on homeschooling within the African American community, with numerous scholars adding to this work. The contributions of various scholars present research that addresses the varying complexities of African American homeschooling. Wellborn (2022) examines the theory, practice, and popular culture of homeschooling Black children in the United States, including how systemic racism often plays a critical role in Black families' decisions to homeschool. Fields-Smith (2020) explores an underrepresented demographic of African American homeschoolers, single Black mothers, and provides a counternarrative to normative ideals on Black mothers, Black education and parental involvement, and African American homeschooling. Puga (2019) offers new insights into how the varying motivations of African American families' decisions to homeschool are often grounded in educational reform and political protest based on the marginalization and hardships many African American families face in traditional education.

Mazama (2016) presents empirical findings regarding African American homeschooling practices, highlighting that Black homeschooled children are primarily provided child-driven learning by their mothers, including knowledge of African American history and culture. Ray (2015) explores the motivations of Black parents to homeschool their children and the academic achievements of their children. Findings indicated that Black parents had similar motivations for homeschooling as any other parents, although the ability to educate their children in African American history and culture played a vital role, and academically, the children tested higher than Black children in public school and equal to or higher than all students in general. Fields-Smith and Kisura (2013) examine homeschooling as resisting the status quo and find that for many Black families, homeschooling is an act of resistance that rescues Black children from the harmful effects and negative consequences of public schooling. Mazama and Lundy (2012) investigate the experiences, views, and actions of Black parents who chose to homeschool and highlight the agency displayed by the parents as they take their children's education into their own hands largely for racial protectionism.

Despite the contributions of these scholars and the evolution of homeschool practices, many beliefs surrounding the phenomenon of homeschooling are homogeneous and limit the scope and possibility of what homeschooling *is* and *can be*, who homeschools, and why families homeschool. Generally, homeschooling is viewed as a practice reserved for White, middle-class, conservation, two-parent households heavily driven by religion and a rejection of "traditional schooling." While the trends mentioned above have a time and place in homeschooling history, the phenomenon has undergone transformation and progression over the years that moves against the static perception of homeschooling. The current view of homeschooling often pushes the idea of "schooling" to the forefront and negates a critical point: the home is and will continue to be a fundamental site for education and learning; schooling and education and learning are not always synonymous. Scholarship continues to offer new insights into homeschooling that move away from and stretch and reframe common homeschooling ideals.

7.2 Moving from Homeschooling Toward Home/Schooling

7.2.1 An Alternative Definition

The term *homeschooling* is generally employed to denote "the routines and habits of schooling in the home" and gives the impression that "children can only learn where there is a hierarchical relationship between teacher and student, and that a systematic set of objectives is necessary to guide the learning process" (Greenwalt, 2019, p. 9). Upon close review of homeschooling literature, variations in defining homeschooling abound. Murphy (2012) presented core definitions of the term provided by scholars over a quarter-century; the years span from 1985 to 2008. While none of the definitions were the same, they all included two key aspects: homeschooling consists of educating a child in the home and is usually done by a parent, guardian, or tutor. People tie the education to "schooling," or an alternative form of education substituted for traditional school. As Murphy (2012) notes, it is evident that homeschoolers are often defined by what they *do not do* instead of what they *do*. Homeschoolers do not spend most of the day in institutionalized settings and do not always have a state-certified teacher providing their instruction. Thus, a popular view is that homeschooling rejects government schooling. Recent scholarship has provided an alternative definition for homeschooling.

In his book, *Home/Schooling: Creating Schools That Work for Kids, Parents, and Teachers,* Greenwalt (2019) introduces a new definition: home/schooling. Home/schooling rejects the premise that children "only learn where there is a hierarchical relationship between teacher and student, and that a systematic set of objectives is necessary to guide the learning endeavor" while still acknowledging that learning is achieved communally (p. 9). Instead, home/schooling "is about rethinking the relationship between home and school, parents and teachers, and even men and women" (Greenwalt, 2019, p. 9). Even when a child attends a traditional or private school, learning and education continue at home. Parents serve as educators or teachers to their children in many areas of life, including schooling. The same parents often questioned regarding their aptitude to educate their children in the home without the supervision of a state-certified teacher would otherwise be parents held responsible for assisting their children with homework and other schooling requirements. Individuals deem the home as where children should learn morals, values, and self-care. The home has always served as a primary site of education and learning in some capacity. Home/schooling involves parents educating their children to more than what is in school textbooks or curriculum; home/schooling involves children being educated to and learning things valued to their parents or families like cultural customs, gardening, cooking, or the importance of family history and connection. Home/schooling involves education integral to a child becoming or living and learning. Education is also the practice of living and learning; children learn from where they live. Home/schooling, therefore, becomes a practice most parents utilize. When referencing the practice adopted by African American families, I will use the term home/schooling from this point forward.

7.2.2 *Rethinking Who Home/Schools*

While one might argue that home/schooling commences in most homes, various families participate in traditional homeschooling. Generally, people view home/schooling as a practice reserved for White, middle-class, conservative Christian, two-parent households. Scholarship has largely contributed to this view. In providing a portrait of the demographics of home/schoolers, Murphy (2012) identified the following characteristics of home/schooling parents: "solidly middle class and financially stable, well-educated, stay-at-home mothers devoted to their families, disproportionately White, married, and Christian" (pp. 16–22). Lois (2013) described the vast majority of home/schoolers as "stay-at-home mothers in two-parent, heterosexual families with husbands supporting the family in the paid labor force" (p. 45). Even in Black families, individuals associate the practice with a two-parent, middle-class, spiritual household (Fields-Smith, 2020). Numerous other scholars (Dwyer & Peters, 2019; Gaither, 2017; Mackey et al., 2011) have provided similar descriptions of the "typical" home/schooling family. However, emerging scholarship is introducing new insight into the diversity of the home/schooling family, especially among African American families.

7.3 African American Home/Schooling

7.3.1 *Current Context for African American Home/Schooling*

In the last decade, there has been an emerging body of scholarship on the motivations of African American home/schoolers, mainly due to the increase of African American families that have opted to home/school. According to Mazama (2016), "the number of homeschooled Black children tripled between 1999 and 2007" (p. 26). By 2013, Black children comprised an estimated 8% of the 2 million homeschooled students (Ray, 2015). As of January 2020, an estimated 2 million children were still being homeschooled in America (HSLDA, 2020). The emergence of the COVID pandemic in March 2020 resulted in an exponential surge in the number of homeschooled children the next school year. There were roughly 3.7 million homeschooled students in the United States in 2020–2021 in grades K-12 (Ray, 2022.). Black students now make up close to 10% of the home/schooling population; it is estimated that over 300,000 Black families home/school. According to the Census Bureau, 3.3% of Black families homeschooled in Spring 2020; by Fall 2020, that number increased to 16% (Eggleston & Fields, 2021). Like their White counterparts, most Black home/schooling families consist of two-parent, married, middle-class households where the mother is identified as the teacher or educator while the father is the primary breadwinner (Mazama, 2016). With more Black families choosing to home/school, some of the families consist of single-parent, low-income households (Fields-Smith, 2020).

The COVID-19 pandemic has introduced another demographic of home/schooling parents: working parents. While there were parents that worked and home/schooled prior to the pandemic, the number of Black parents that opted to continue home/schooling once schools reopened increased exponentially. Reilly (2022) notes that while the pandemic served as a catalyst for many Black parents to begin or continue home/schooling, the decision was driven by varying motivations, with control of their children's education being salient. Black parents taking control of their children's education is nothing new. Historically, African Americans have gone to great lengths to educate themselves and extend that education to the Black community. Black families have demonstrated communal efforts and agency to share knowledge, teach one another, and resist the oppressive forces emplaced to refuse and limit educational opportunity with an "any means necessary" mentality (Fields-Smith; 2020). Present-day Black families taking ownership of their children's schooling extends the "any means necessary" mentality and continues a legacy of educational resilience traditionally displayed in African American efforts to overcome numerous hardships and pursue educational freedom and excellence.

7.3.2 *African American Home/Schooling: Continuing a Legacy of Educational Resilience*

Resilience is inherent to the history of African Americans. In addition to facing numerous forms of oppression, marginalization, and dehumanization, African Americans have fought for civil and human rights easily obtained by others. The right to education has been a constant battle for most Black and Brown people. Traditionally, when education has been denied and restricted, African Americans resisted and persisted by using any means to educate themselves and their children. As a result, educational resilience became a staple of Black people and families. Education resilience is the ability to have positive education outcomes despite facing significant adversity (Cunningham & Swanson, 2010). Self-taughtness became salient to African American education (Williams, 2009). The notion of self-taughtness is rooted in the long-standing history of African Americans' communal efforts and agency to learn and teach one another by any means necessary. Enslaved Africans first fostered self-taughtness; agency and self-determination were imperative to learn to read and establish schools for themselves (Fields-Smith, 2020). Enslaved people valued education, particularly literacy, because it provided access to information, ideas, news, and for many, survival and freedom. Therefore, self-taughtness was cultivated and adopted in many creative manners. Bartering and trading skills, money, and food for spelling lessons, words, or letters were one way some enslaved people gained literacy. Some enslaved people turned to their master's children or other white children to learn what the children had learned at school each day. Many enslaved mothers encouraged their children to "play school" with their master's children. Some enslaved people used caves or pit schools, large pits dug up deep in the woods and covered with shrubs and bushes, as sites to teach one another (Williams, 2009). There is evidence of some enslaved people adopting home/schooling as a means of teaching their children and encouraging self-taughtness.

In the book, *Self-Taught: African American Education in Slavery and Freedom*, Williams (2009) highlights an instance where an enslaved woman used a form of "home/schooling" to educate her children. Williams (2009) tells the story of Mattie Jackson. Jackson and her mother, Ellen Turner, and brothers and sisters were sold into slavery. Turner worked to educate her daughter in various ways, which resulted in Jackson learning to read and write. According to Williams (2009),

> Becoming literate required them to employ creative tactics. Jackson does not reveal how her mother learned to read, but presumably, the mother taught her daughter at night in their room in the Lewis home. Accounts of such efforts make it evident that even in slavery, with its violence, insults, and punishing labor, many African Americans yearned to become literate and access the news and ideas that otherwise would have been beyond their reach. (p. 12)

Turner's efforts to create a learning environment within the Lewis home and educate her daughter in literacy and survival tactics resulted in Jackson seeking and becoming a free woman. Similarly, King (2011) provides other examples of enslaved people using home/schooling to educate their children. As Greenwalt (2019) posited, home/schooling always has been more than textbook education; it includes education on how to live, learn, flourish, and survive. Enslaved people considered "smart" children as ones who learned acceptable behavior that kept them from reprisal or punishment by enslavers. "Smart" children learned to be mannerable and respectful to their elders. In pursuit of protection, many enslaved people used home/schooling to teach their children how to maneuver through slavery and southern etiquette and expectations, survival tactics needed to pursue literacy and more academic education. As King (2011) notes:

> Both real and fictive kinfolk seized every opportunity to teach children how to forge a balance between social courtesy to others and their self-esteem. The urgency of the matter was ever-present, whether during the rigorous period between sunup and sundown or after dark in their quarters. Evenings were special times to educate and entertain; children often learned adages constructed to advise them and raise their consciousness. "What goes around comes around," "Beauty is only skin deep, but love is to the bone," and "The blacker the berry, the sweeter the juice" are but a few of the maxims that cautioned children against capriciousness and at the same time instilled confidence about coloration in a society where pigmentation mattered. At the end of the day, while in their cabins, children learned about their culture from older Africans or their descendants, who passed recollections from one generation to another in keeping with their oral traditions. (p. 175)

Stories like Jackson's (Williams, 2009) and King's (2011) highlight how the practice of home/schooling is not new to Black parents and is rooted in a long history of educational resilience. The historical practice of self-taughtness fostered by African American ancestors still informs the present practice of Black parents to take ownership of their children's education and teach them by any means necessary.

7.4 Implications

7.4.1 Implications for Understanding Family Resilience

Educational resilience remains imperative to African Americans' quest for education. While education is no longer illegal for African Americans, problems still exist in it being inequitable, oppressive, and marginalizing, especially within the public school systems. As noted by the *Black Girls Matter: Pushed Out, Overpoliced, and Underprotected* report, schools across the country are using punitive disciplinary measures and policies to surveillance, punish, expel, and criminalize girls of color, particularly African American girls (Crenshaw et al., 2015). Crenshaw et al. (2015) note that a study revealed that teachers stated they use disciplinary measures exercised against African American girls to "encourage them to adopt more 'acceptable' qualities of femininity, such as being quieter and more passive" (p. 24). Students of color are overrepresented in special education, experience greater segregation and worse outcomes, and receive suspensions at a higher rate. Suspensions are highest among students of color with individualized education plans (IEPs) with or without disabilities (Morgan, 2020). A review of African American home/schooling literature from 1996 to 2015 highlighted four major themes contributing to Black parents'motivation to home/school: disproportionate discipline within public schools, lack of sociocultural connection in curriculum and teaching style, low academic expectations, and concerns of safety. Home/schooling fosters family resilience by allowing Black parents to resist oppressive and harmful practices instituted by public education while taking ownership of their children's education in a space that offers educational freedoms and greater possibilities.

7.4.2 *Implications for Practice*

7.4.2.1 Educational Resilience and Academic Freedom

Home/schooling allows parents to cater learning specific to their children, especially children with embodied learning conditions that may require specialized instruction methods or children who show promise of excelling at a greater rate (Dywer & Peters, 2019; Murphy, 2012). There are academic factors that lead to many Black families home/schooling. Dissatisfaction and distrust with public school instruction result in many parents and caregivers opting to educate their children at home. Curriculum and content are an issue for many parents, and home/schooling provides parents the freedom to create or purchase a curriculum of choice (Murphy, 2012). Some families choose to gravitate toward unschooling and employ child-driven learning, which allows children to follow their interests (Mazama, 2016). As a result, children are more involved with what they learn and how they learn. Ultimately, home/schooling offers Black parents a means to diversify learning for their children and incorporate a fluid structure that involves learning culturally and historically relevant content in diverse spaces and with different instructional tools.

7.4.2.2 Prioritization of Family

Home/schooling permits Black families to spend time and learn and grow together. Lois (2013) notes that home/schooling provides a means for many mothers to devote more time to nurturing their children while they are young. Many parents value extended time with their children and view home/schooling as a way to enhance family relationships (Murphy, 2012). For some Black families, home/schooling is rooted in the tradition of homeplace (Fields-Smith, 2020). bell hooks' concept of homeplace draws on the critical role of Black women in the home and community historically. It emphasizes Black women's role in making the home a critical site of resistance against injustice and instead a site of love, power, and edification (Fields-Smith, 2020; Fields-Smith & Kisura, 2013). In her essay, "Homeplace (a Site of Resistance)," hooks (1997) states:

> Black women resisted by making homes where all black people could strive to be subjects, not objects, where we could be affirmed in our minds and hearts despite poverty, hardship, and deprivation, where we could restore to ourselves the dignity denied us on the outside of the public world. (p. 384)

In creating homeplace, Black women construct a space of safety and opportunity that nurtures growth and healing, especially from racist domination (hooks, 1997). Home/schooling allows Black families to create spaces where their children can be educated and thrive in a culture with people with whom they share love and interests.

7.4.2.3 Racial Protectionism

Home/schooling addresses the concerns of equitable education for some Black families. For many families with concerns over racial disparity, negative stereotypes, lack of cultural and historical representation, insufficient school funding, and inequitable learning conditions, home/schooling has been an empowering alternative to the status quo (Dywer & Peters, 2019; Mazama & Lundy, 2012; Puga, 2019; Ray, 2015). Mazama and Lundy (2012) introduced the term racial protectionist to identify "Black parents who have opted to educate their offspring at home at least in part in an attempt to shield their children from the racism they have experienced in school or that they do not wish their children to be subjected to" (p. 733). For many Black families, home/schooling is an act of resistance and protest against oppressive forces that hinder productive learning and cause emotional harm. I painted *At Home, Resisting!* (See Fig. 7.1) to pay homage to and celebrate black parents, especially black mothers, resisting normative and inequitable educational practices by electing to home/school. My husband and I began our home/schooling journey with our two sons a decade ago. We were both very knowledgeable of the racial disparity that Black children often face in schools. Our apprehension over institutions like the school to prison pipeline and the funneling of Black children into special education made the decision to home/school easy for us. While educating our boys was of extreme importance, protecting them from spirit murdering was just as important. Spirit murdering is the use of disciplinary practices, racism, prejudice, marginalization, or negative attitudes by teachers or school administrators on children that result in broken spirits. Spirit murdering can be pedagogical, institutional, or individual and occurs daily for many Black children in classrooms (Fields-Smith, 2020). Home/schooling allows many Black parents to affirm and embolden their children's learning and education. Additionally, Fields-Smith (2020) offers a new consideration and motivation for home/schooling: healing. The author notes that Black parents generally express their desire to home/school as a pathway to healing from the racial disparities and discrimination they or their children experience with traditional schools.

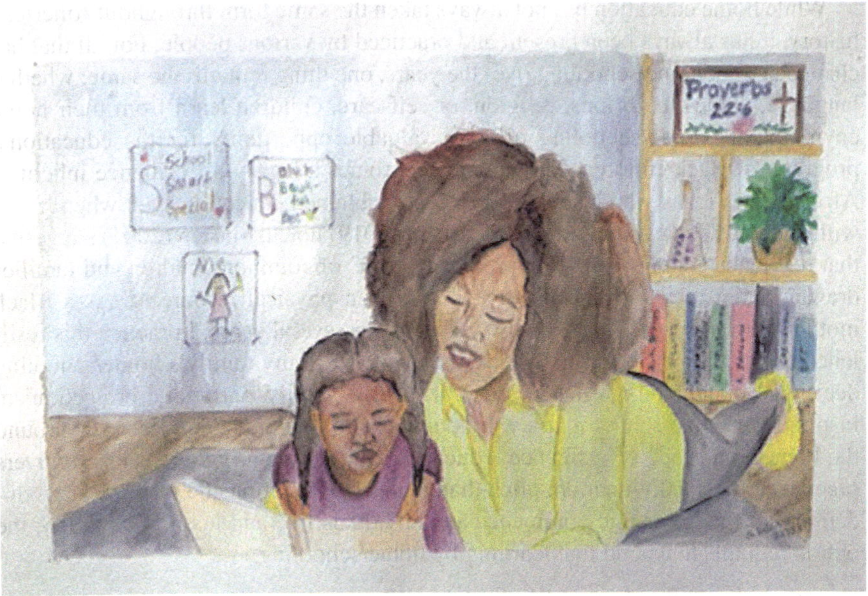

Fig. 7.1 Stacie Warner (2020) At Home, Resisting! [watercolor] Oklahoma City, Oklahoma

7.5 Conclusion

With the recent surge in the number of home/schooled Black children, new discussions, beliefs, and historical markers about this multidimensional practice are emerging. There are philosophical debates that home/schooling is either inherently bad or always good. Homeschool critics argue that home/schooling is inherently "bad" for the whole of a child. In their view, home/schooling presents deficiencies in students' education and values and should have strict guidelines and mandates. As Dywer and Peters (2019) point out, no one has created a standard of "bad" and demonstrated how homeschooling presents deficiencies to fall below that standard. The capacious nature of home/schooling makes the view of it being inherently "bad" challenging to argue. Home/school advocates view homeschooling as a superior option for schooling and tend to believe home/schooling should not be state governed (Dywer & Peters, 2019). Many advocates believe that home/schools are better than public or private schools. As asserted by Dywer and Peters (2019), to argue that home/schooling is "all" good "...would have to rest on the belief that whatever any parents do with their children is ipso facto good for the children" (p. 115). Such an argument is both unfathomable and illogical. Home/schooling has strengths and weaknesses, much like public or private schooling. It works exceptionally well for some families and lends itself to being the best option for their circumstances. Historically, it has served the interests of African American families attempting to resist oppressive circumstances, overcome challenges associated with "traditional" education, and gain educational autonomy.

While home education has not always taken the same form throughout American history, it has always been present and practiced by various people. For all that has changed about home/schooling over the years, one thing remains the same: whether language, values, traditions, religion, or self-care, children learn from their home environment. Home/schooling offers a valuable opportunity for the educational progress of Black children. The practice continues a legacy of resilience inherit to African Americans who have persevered and obtained education even when it was withheld and illegal to pursue. As Anderson (2019) notes, Masten (2001) suggested that resilience "comes from the 'ordinary magic' of common children and families drawing from their emotional, mental, and even physical resources." As a Black mother who has home/schooled my two sons for several years, I practice this resilience firsthand. While spirituality has been salient in my family's home/schooling decision, educational resilience, prioritization of family, and racial protectionism inspired our home/school journey. It is time to reframe the beliefs centered around the home as a space of resilience, education, and learning. Parents and caregivers practice home/schooling more often than realized. Education and learning are foundational to the home and commence as individuals live and learn. Thankfully, the option remains to extend that learning by home/schooling.

Questions for Thought and Discussion

1. What implications might a continued rise in the number of Black families that chose home/schooling over traditional schooling have on education? Society?
2. An emerging body of scholarship exploring African American home/schooling has been growing since 2014. What is the significance of studying the phenomenon of African American home/schooling?
3. Should parents have to meet certain qualifications (i.e., educational, professional) to home/school their child(ren)? Why or why not?
4. Given the present state of the COVID-19 pandemic and its impact on society and education, should schools give more consideration to the potential of collaborative home education between parents and schools?
5. What would it look like for educators and educational institutions to lean into the notion of schooling as a shared vocation practiced by them and the family, in a manner that is less hierarchical and more complementary?

Conflict of Interest I have no known conflict of interest to disclose

References

Anderson, L. A. (2019). Rethinking resilience theory in African American families: Fostering positive adaptations and transformative social justice. *Journal of Family Theory & Review, 11*(3), 385–397. https://doi.org/10.1111/jftr.12343

Cremin, L. A. (1970). *American education, the colonial experience, 1607–1783*. Harper & Row.

Crenshaw, K. W., Ocen, P., & Nanda, J. (2015). Black girls matter: Pushed out, overpoliced and underprotected.

Cunningham, M., & Swanson, D. P. (2010). Educational resilience in African American adolescents. *The Journal of Negro Education*, 473–487.

Dwyer, J. G., & Peters, S. F. (2019). *Homeschooling: The history and philosophy of a controversial practice*. The University of Chicago Press.

Eggleston, C., & Fields, J. (2021). *Census bureau's Household Pulse Survey shows significant increase in homeschooling rates in fall 2020*. Census.gov. https://www.census.gov/library/stories/2021/03/homeschooling-on-the-rise-during-covid-19-pandemic.html

Ferguson, A. A. (2020). *Bad boys: Public schools in the making of black masculinity*. University of Michigan Press.

Fields-Smith, C. (2020). *Exploring single Black mothers' resistance through homeschooling*. Palgrave Macmillan.

Fields-Smith, C., & Kisura, M. W. (2013). Resisting the status quo: The narratives of Black homeschoolers in metro-Atlanta and metro-DC. *Peabody Journal of Education, 88*(3), 265–283. https://doi.org/10.1080/0161956x.2013.796823

Gaither, M. (2017). *Homeschool: An American history*. Palgrave Macmillan.

Greenwalt, K. (2019). *Home/schooling: Creating schools that work for kids, parents and teachers*. Brill.

hooks, B. (1997). Homeplace: A site of resistance. In Undoing place? A geographical reader (pp. 33–38). Routledge.

Hslda. (2020). What is homeschooling and how does it work? Retrieved April 29, 2020, from https://hslda.org/post/what-is-homeschooling

Ingold, T. (2017, April 26). Anthropology and/as education. *The Education and Social Research Institute's (ESRI) Blog*. http://www.esriblog.info/esri-seminar-professor-tim-ingold-anthropology-andas-education

Ingold, T. (2018). *Anthropology and/as education*. Routledge.

King, W. (2011). Stolen childhood: Slave youth in nineteenth-century America. Indiana University Press.

Lawrence, A. (2019). Precolonial Indigenous education in the western hemisphere and Pacific.

Lois, J. (2013). *Home is where the school is: The logic of homeschooling and the emotional labor of mothering*. New York University Press.

Mackey, B. W., Reese, K., & Mackey, W. C. (2011). Demographics of home schoolers: A regional analysis within the national parameters. *Education, 132*(1), 133–140.

Masten, A. S. (2001). Ordinary magic: Resilience processes in development. *American Psychologist, 56*(3), 227–238. https://doi.org/10.1037/0003-066X.56.3.227

Mazama, A. (2016). African American homeschooling practices: Empirical evidence. *Theory and Research in Education, 14*(1), 26–44. https://doi.org/10.1177/1477878515615734

Mazama, A., & Lundy, G. (2012). African American homeschooling as racial protectionism. *Journal of Black Studies, 43*(7), 723–748. https://doi.org/10.1177/0021934712457042

Morgan, H. (2020). Misunderstood and mistreated: Students of color in special education. *Online Submission, 3*(2), 71–81.

Murphy, J. (2012). *Homeschooling in America: Capturing and assessing the Movement*. SkyHorse Pub.

Puga, L. (2019). "Homeschooling is our protest:" Educational liberation for African American homeschooling families in Philadelphia, PA. *Peabody Journal of Education, 94*(3), 281–296. https://doi.org/10.1080/0161956X.2019.1617579

Ray, B. D. (2015). The social and emotional health of homeschooled students in the united states: A population-based comparison with publicly schooled students based on the national survey of children's health, 2007. *Home School Researcher, 31*(1). https://www.nheri.org/home-school-researcher-the-social-and-emotional-health-of-homeschooled-students-in-the-united-states-a-population-based-comparison-with-publicly-schooled-students-based-on-the-national-survey-of-child/

Ray, B. D. (2022). *How many homeschool students are there in the United States? Pre-COVID-19 and post-COVID-19: New data*. National Home Education Research Institute. https://www.nheri.org/how-many-homeschool-students-are-there-in-the-united-states-pre-covid-19-and-post-covid-19/

Reilly, K. (2022, February 28). *Homeschooling has become more popular among black families.* Time. https://time.com/6151375/black-families-homeschooling/

Urban, W. J., Wagoner, J. L., & Gaither, M. (2019). *American education: A history*. Routledge, Taylor & Francis.

Walsh, F. (2016). Applying a family resilience framework in training, practice, and research: Mastering the art of the possible. *Family Process, 55*(4), 616–632. https://doi.org/10.1111/famp.12260

Wellborn, C. (2022). Homeschooling black children in the US: Theory, Practice, and Popular Culture: edited by Khadijah Ali-Coleman and Cheryl Fields-Smith (Eds.). (2022). Cambridge, MA: Information Age Publishing, 242 pp., $45.99 (paperback), ISBN 978-1648027826.

Williams, H. A. (2009). *Self-taught: African American education in slavery and freedom.* University of North Carolina Press.

Chapter 8
Resilience and Black Identity Considerations for Black Mental Health Research

LaRicka R. Wingate, Vanessa Oliphant, Déjà N. Clement, and Olufunke Benson

Black people have endured centuries of oppression, violent abuse, and attempted erasure from history (Hadden, 2003; Hartman, 2008; Kambon, 2012; Hine, 2007), and the field of psychology has historically ignored this oppression by primarily producing deficit-based psychological research concerning Black people. European conceptualizations of Black behavior were limited, and the earlier writings on Black people argue that they are deficient, inferior, and pathologized. This work did not acknowledge the fact that Black people were able to survive and thrive despite the regular oppression that they faced. However, it is clear that the early writings of Black psychologists came from a more positive psychologically oriented perspective. A seminal article by Joseph White (1970), "Toward a Black Psychology," articulated a wellness and non-deficit-based psychology for Black people. White (1970) argued that it was impossible to study Black people with theories and concepts that were created for white people by white people. He explained that this led to many false, inaccurate, and incomplete conclusions. White (1970) also explicitly argued for a discipline of psychology that takes into consideration historical context, challenges Eurocentric ideologies about Blackness, and intentionally uses a non-deficit-based conceptualization when examining the psychological experiences of Black people (Cokley et al., 2019). White's (1970) seminal article essentially spawned a new revolution of psychology (i.e., Black Psychology) that aimed to humanize the mental health of African/Black people, while producing culturally relevant psychological research from an African-centered worldview.

An African-centered worldview can be described as a set of principles, values, and belief systems grounded in African traditions and informed by indigenous African healing practices that honors the connection between the mind, body, and

L. R. Wingate (✉) · V. Oliphant · D. N. Clement · O. Benson
Department of Psychology, Oklahoma State University, Stillwater, OK, USA
e-mail: laricka.wingate@okstate.edu

J. M. Koch et al. (eds.), *Identity as Resilience in Minoritized Communities*, Emerging Issues in Family and Individual Resilience,
https://doi.org/10.1007/978-3-031-38977-1_8

spirit (Ojelade et al., 2014). The field of Black psychology, as well as Africana studies, have been pivotal in advancing theory, research, and interventions from an African-centered worldview (Caroll, 2010).

Scholars trained in the discipline of Black psychology have dedicated their careers to developing research and creating therapeutic techniques that embody the principles found within an African-centered worldview (Belgrave & Allison, 2014; James Myers et al., 2022, Kambon, 2012), such as an emphasis on harmony and oneness, collectivism, survival of the group and spirituality. In this chapter, the conceptualization of Black wellness and resilience will be primarily grounded in an African-centered worldview, which is commonly emphasized within the field of Black psychology.

Scholars in the field of Black psychology describe wellness from an African-centered holistic perspective. Essentially, wellness occurs when there is a symbiotic connection between the mind, body, and spirit (Phillips, 1990; Tsa-Tsala, 1997). In order to talk about Black resilience, we must discuss Black well-being. There is a reciprocal relationship between wellness and resilience. For one to be well, every aspect of a person must be acknowledged, nurtured, and supported. Being well is intimately connected to being resilient. Although some scholars conceptualize resilience as the ability to overcome challenges (Goldstein & Brooks, 2013), resilience needs to be more than this for Black people. Resilience for Black people should also include the intentional prioritization of psychological health, physical preservation, and emotional stability after overcoming challenges. An emphasis on wellness rather than the ability to overcome situations (i.e., resilience) acknowledges that a person's well-being must be nurtured following challenging circumstances. The intentional act of caring for oneself after undergoing difficult occurrences is engaging in well-being and resilience behaviors and is in direct alignment with an African-centered worldview. When conceptualizing resilience for Black people, it is also important to consider the overall humanity of and the history of this population because it illuminates why preservation and wellness is an integral part of resilience.

There is an interdependent relationship between the mind, body, and spirit (Phillips, 1990; Tsala-Tsala, 1997), and prior research has explicitly identified several associations between the mind and the body. For instance, symptoms relating to depression and anxiety are commonly linked to medically unexplained health conditions such as irritable bowel syndrome, fibromyalgia, and chronic pelvic pain (Arnold et al., 2007; Lydiard, 2001; Miller-Matero et al., 2016; Prince et al., 2007). One study indicated that 15% of patients seen in primary care have medically unexplained somatic symptoms often attributed to mental health disorders such as depression and anxiety (Prince et al., 2007). Other studies have found that 50% of cancer patients suffered from depression or anxiety (Massie, 2004) and patients with type II diabetes were twice as likely to experience depression (Gonzalez et al., 2008).

Research in the sub-discipline of Positive psychology (Seligman, 2002) has also identified the connection between mental and physical health. Positive psychology specifically suggests that an optimistic perspective on life can be connected to better physical health outcomes, which can play a vital role in one's overall well-being and resiliency. For instance, numerous studies have indicated positive physical health outcomes related to the psychological constructs of gratitude and hope (Krause et al., 2017; Legler et al., 2019; Scioli et al., 2016; Snyder, 2004). One study found that stronger feelings of gratitude are related to lower levels of HbA1c, which is an indicator of blood sugar control (Krause et al., 2017). Another study found that gratitude may be linked to cardiac health and recovery (Legler et al., 2019). In a survey of oncologists, hope was considered an important psychological factor contributing to mortality (Cousins, 1989). Essentially, previous research confirms there is a link between physical and mental health, which further supports the argument that nurturing the relationship between the mind, body, and spirit can better equip Black people to fully engage in resilience.

8.1 Black Wellness and Black-Specific Coping

Research in the field of Black psychology suggest that utilizing culturally specific ways of coping and endorsing affirmative and validating pro-Black attitudes (i.e., racial identity) can impact Black people's psychological well-being (Constantine et al., 2002; Lewis-Coles & Constantine, 2006; Pyant & Yanico, 1991; Sellers et al., 2006; Wilson et al., 2017). To measure culturally specific ways of coping, Utsey et al. (2000) created the Africultural Coping Systems Inventory (ACSI). In this measure there are four subscales: (a) cognitive and emotional debriefing, adaptive reactions to stressors; (b) collective coping, finding comfort from social connections; (c) spiritual-centered coping, dependence on a higher power and/or one's religious practice, and (d) ritual-centered coping, reliance on the use of rituals (Utsey et al., 2000).

One study using the ACSI measure found that African American women were more likely to use spirituality and collective ways of coping when dealing with racism-related stressors (Lewis-Coles & Constantine, 2006). Another study showed that African American adolescents utilized collective and spiritual ways of coping when dealing with stressful situations (Constantine et al., 2002). Other studies found that Africultural coping strategies can serve as a buffer against suicidal ideation for African American female college students (Morrison & Hopkins, 2019). In a study that assessed intimate partner violence (IPV) and existential well-being for African American women (Hampton-Anderson et al., 2022), researchers found that spiritual and ritual-centered coping may serve as potential protective factor against IPV. Additionally, culture-specific coping and spiritual well-being were found to be significant predictors of quality of life (Utsey et al., 2007); and spiritual coping techniques have been found to help manage COVID-19-related chronic stress and trauma (le Roux et al., 2022). While professional mental health support may not always be easily assessable, Black people have ingrained cultural resources in their communities that can aid in supporting their mental health such as the use of spirituality, social support, rituals, and individual debriefing strategies (Kambon, 2012; Utsey et al., 2000, 2007).

8.2 Black Wellness and Racial Identity

Intentionally finding ways to increase the endorsement of affirmative pro-Black attitudes is one approach for positively supporting Black people's well-being and centering resilience. In the field of Black psychology, researchers have described the endorsement of affirmative and validating pro-Black attitudes as racial identity (Gibson et al., 2022; Pyant & Yanico). Racial identity is the significance that African Americans place on race when describing themselves (Sellers et al., 2006). Numerous studies have found a positive relationship between higher levels of racial identity and overall psychological well-being for African Americans (Gibson et al., 2022; Pyant & Yanico, 1991; Sellers et al., 2006; Wilson et al., 2017). Black people with higher levels of racial identity tend to view their race as more central to their self-definition and have a sense of connectedness to their racial group (Yip et al., 2006). Studies have found that racial identity attitudes are protective against the effect of race-related stress on mental health (Jones et al., 2007) and racial identity can moderate the relationship between discrimination and depressive symptoms (Banks & Kohn-Wood, 2007). Another study found that racial identity was a predictor of African American's academic performance (Rowley et al., 1998).

While a traditional psychological approach may not focus on racial identity as an effective treatment option, a strong racial identity is needed to survive in a society that constantly promotes implicit and explicit messaging around Black people's worth, beauty, and intellectual ability. Frequently witnessing Black people die at the hands of police, inadequate access to healthcare and education, and pervasive poverty can negatively impact the psychological well-being of Black people (Alang, 2019; Do et al., 2019; Hawkins, 2022; Staggers-Hakim, 2016; Tynes et al., 2019). As a result, it is imperative to intentionally find ways to increase Black people's racial identity to positively support their well-being and overall resilience. Collectively, this research highlights the positive impact that strong racial identity has in bolstering resilience and subsequently improving health and wellness in Black communities. Creating affirming spaces and opportunities that support the unique identities of Black individuals, communities, and families is central to creating positive health outcomes. While this research demonstrates that racial identity is a key component of building resilience, the unique and complex identities that Black communities hold expand beyond race. These unique and complex identities are often seen as a deficit as they intersect with compounding systems of oppression, yet research has not yet examined how these complex identities may foster resilience.

8.3 The Integration of Resilience and Intersectionality: Through the Lens of an Intersectional Socio-ecological Model

Historical and continuing racism and systemic oppression have had a multilevel (i.e., individual, community, societal, economical) impact on the United States. Notably, racial health disparities are associated with significant economic deficits including $35 billion in excess healthcare expenditures, $10 billion in illness-related lost productivity, and approximately $200 billion in premature deaths (LaVeist et al., 2011). As research on systemic racism and oppression expands in the fields of psychology and behavioral science, there becomes a growing need to identify resilience factors that may mitigate the impact of racism on Black communities and families. While psychological research has primarily focused on individual-level factors, the continuation of racism and systemic oppression in the United States have been deemed a public health crisis that expands beyond the individual (Vandiver, 2020). Therefore, to develop interventions and preventative strategies to combat racism and systemic oppression, it is imperative that resilience researchers and scholars examine resilience at intersectional and structural levels.

The integration of intersectionality and the socio-ecological model allows researchers to explore the variability of resilience that occurs at individual, community, and structural levels which may lead to different, but not deficient, outcomes. We propose a paradigm shift toward a more holistic, intersectional, and cultural model of resilience research in Black communities. We propose a theoretical model that merges the socio-ecological model (Bronfenbrenner, 1979), resiliency theory (Fergus & Zimmerman, 2005), and intersectionality (Crenshaw, 1989) to guide future research (see Fig. 8.1). Specifically, we are interested in the various individual and societal systems in which Black individuals, families, and communities intersect, and how those systems positively affect psychological and physical health outcomes to generate resilience.

Psychology and public health researchers can work to bolster systems that promote resilience through research that aims to develop systemic facilitation intervention strategies that mitigate harm from discrimination and health disparities across ecological levels. The socio-ecological model (Bronfenbrenner, 1979) explicitly acknowledges the ways in which various layers of an individual's environment can affect their development and functioning. The initial theory considers the intersecting layers embedded within that environment, including an individual level within micro-, meso-, exo-, and macro-systems (Bronfenbrenner, 1979). As research has continued on the socio-ecological model, these systems have been simplified to describe individual, interpersonal, organizational, community, and policy factors that may promote or harm an individual's health outcomes and behaviors (Kilanowski, 2017; Watson-Thompson et al., 2022). The individual level describes the unique statuses of power, privilege, and identity of an individual (e.g., race, gender, individual attitudes, beliefs, behaviors). Previous research that has used the socio-ecological model to describe resilience has taken a deficit and singular

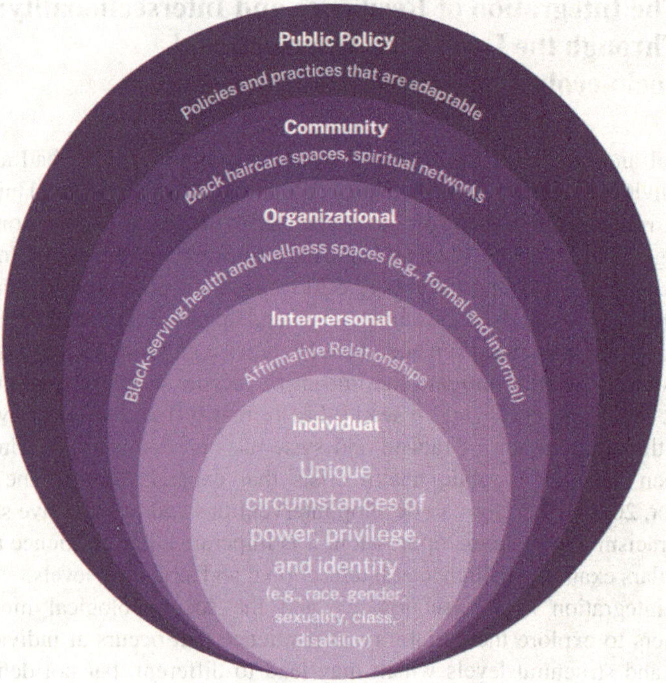

Fig. 8.1 A resilience-based, intersectional, socio-ecological model

approach to identity (i.e., considering the multiple marginalized identities of youth as single-issue risk factors) rather than a strengths-based approach. In the proposed model, we take an intersectional and strengths-based approach to understanding identity. For example, an individual who has a strong sense and confidence in their multiple unique statuses of power, privilege, and identity (e.g., a strong racial identity and gender identity) may be more resilient than an individual with a lower sense of identity. The interpersonal level describes close relationships and interactions an individual holds (e.g., family, peers, coworkers; Bronfenbrenner, 1979). In the proposed model, this may include having relationships that provide affirmative experiences and opportunities that support an individual's intersectional identities (e.g., strong relationships with friends, family, peers). The organizational level describes factors related to access and equity within the physical environment that bolster resilience (e.g., having access to mental health support within schools; healthcare facilities and professionals that are culturally responsive and affirmative). The community level describes relationships among organizations and to resources that bolster resilience such as spiritual networks, schools, and support groups. Finally, the policy and practice level focuses on the values and beliefs of the larger culture within which these other systems are embedded (Bronfenbrenner, 1988). These systems may seem separate; however, they are inextricably linked. The interactions, or transactions, between these systems can help to explain much of the complexity in the lived experiences of Black individuals. To the authors' knowledge, there are little to no studies that explicitly examine the socio-ecological model in the context of resilience and positive health outcomes for Black individuals and communities. The socio-ecological model provides a good foundation for promoting resilience by offering insight into how resilience may occur across different levels which can lead to wellness for Black communities. Our proposed model aims to build on the socio-ecological model by using a strengths-based approach and highlighting the intersections and compounding positive impact of these systems that may promote resilience (see Fig. 8.1).

Resiliency theory states that there are context-specific factors that can promote either resilience or risk among individuals who face adversity (Fergus & Zimmerman, 2005). More recently, research has expanded to explore structural/systemic factors that either bolster or harm resilience and individual adaptations in the face of systems of oppression (Shaw et al., 2016). We define intersectional resilience as the unique strengths that individuals with multiple marginalized statuses, communities, and structural systems possess that may produce a protective effect that mitigates adversity and promotes wellness. While there is extensive research that highlights the negative and chronic impact of racism on mental and physical health, there is less research that applies resilience theory to understand the strengths and protective factors that mitigate racial gaps in health. Identifying strengths and protective factors in multilevel and structural contexts allows researchers to identify and understand possibilities to promote more positive outcomes. Within Black populations, research has demonstrated that greater resilience can improve cognitive health (McDonough et al., 2022), cardiovascular health (Kim et al., 2020), mental health (Boyd et al., 2022; Catabay et al., 2019), and sexual health (Buttram, 2019; Follins et al., 2014). Many Black families and communities have important strengths that foster resilience and can mitigate the impact of systemic racism and oppression. Murry et al. (2022) and Stern et al. (2022) both discuss integrative models of attachment and stress which help to understand how racialized stressors may impact the parent-child relationship in Black families but also how Black families develop self-regulation, attachment security, and social-emotional competencies to develop resilience. Specifically, Murry and colleagues highlight that experiences of racial discrimination have a significant, negative, and long-term impact on parent-child relationships and psychological functioning. However, exposure to discrimination during childhood is associated with increased social competence and decreased symptoms of depression in adolescence (Murry et al., 2022). Further, Stern et al. (2022) call for increased research that aims to "decolonize" and integrate a multilevel approach to implementing anti-racist cultural perspectives into research that examines parent-child relationships in Black families. They highlight how different aspects of culture help to foster resilience outcomes in Black families that may help to address inequities within health outcomes but also improve policy and practice for Black families. Collectively, this research highlights that psychological research has many gaps in understanding how resilience is developed and maintained in Black communities. In discussing the future of research on racism and health, Neblett (2019) calls for increased research that aims to understand the complexity of resilience and racial health disparities. Specifically, they highlight that resilience should not be solely conceptualized at the individual level, as we know that community plays a huge role. They also state that examining resilience from a multilevel perspective may aid in the development of improved culturally informed interventions and subsequent health outcomes (Neblett, 2019). Further research and theory are needed to understand Black community resilience and how this occurs across multiple levels of systems.

Research demonstrates that community interventions have been effective in reducing poor mental and physical health outcomes among Black adults, youth, and families. Research has highlighted the positive impact of Africultural-centered community interventions that center the importance and cultural significance of informal helping networks found within haircare spaces in the Black community. Community interventions situated within Black haircare spaces have been associated with developing positive mental and physical health outcomes (Lateef et al., 2022). Mbilishaka (2018a, b) developed "Psychohairapy – A community health model created to secure space for Black women to address mental health and well-being." Research on "Psychohairapy" demonstrates that hair care in Black womanhood is deeply rooted in tradition, culture, and community which allows for Black hair care professionals to be able to provide a community space that fosters resilience. Psychohairapy has been associated with greater psychological wellness among Black women (Mbilishaka, 2018a, b) and Black men (Mbilishaka et al., 2021). Community interventions using Black barbershops have been associated with improved hypertension (Victor et al., 2011), mental health outcomes in Black men (Curry et al., 2022), and early childhood mental health in Black children. Another community intervention that explores the impact of Black community on psychological and physical well-being is Sister circles – Black women-focused community groups that provide culturally informed support, education, and resources for mental and physical health (Neal-Barnett et al., 2011). Sister circles have been demonstrated to be effective in reducing anxiety, improving diet, improving stress management, and increasing health literacy (Gaston et al., 2007; Neal-Barnett et al., 2011). Lastly, while these community-level interventions have been associated with positive mental health outcomes, research is still limited in the integration of various intersectional factors that could strengthen these interventions. Research on resilience in Black communities often highlights that no factor alone (i.e., individual, community, or societal) creates this path of resilience to positive outcomes, rather the intersection of these factors fosters greater resilience.

Rooted in Black Feminist thought and the work of the Combahee River Collective, the language of intersectionality has been used to describe the interlocking systems of oppression rooted in racism and sexism (Collective, 1983; Collins, 1986). The term intersectionality was coined by Kimberlé Crenshaw, a lawyer and African American feminist scholar, as she witnessed Black women experiencing harsher outcomes when navigating the workforce and criminal justice system due to their racial and gender identities (Crenshaw, 1989). Since then, intersectionality has become a concept in social science and health research that addresses how multiple aspects of identity such as race, class, gender, or ability intersect in different contexts and systems over time to produce inequity (Case, 2013; Cho et al., 2013; Warner & Shields, 2013). Intersectionality describes the oppression structurally produced and simultaneously experienced by individuals through and across diverse social categories of identity and aims to address social inequities based on highlighting and disrupting positions of privilege and power (Hankivsky et al., 2014). Further, as a theory of power relations, an intersectional approach aims to explore interlocking unjust power dynamics and considers how these categories simultaneously affect peoples' lives (Cole, 2009; Crenshshaw, 1989). Similar to the socio-ecological model, authors have highlighted the importance of incorporating intersectionality into resilience research and frameworks (Neblett, 2019).

8.4 Intersectional Resilience Model

Although an intersectional framework has been useful in highlighting systems of power, privilege, and oppression, and posing critical insights about the overlapping social categories of identity (Crenshshaw, 1989; Hankivsky et al., 2014), to date, researchers have not explored how this framework may provide insight on positive aspects of power or identity interactions, in addition to community-level interactions that boost resilience in Black individuals and communities. However, there has been a collection of recent studies that have examined the relationship between intersectionality and resilience in other marginalized communities. Parmenter et al. (2021) discuss taking an intersectional approach to understanding inequities that exist for LGBTQ people of color in accessing community resilience resources (e.g., support groups, organizations, culturally responsive and trauma-informed mentors). They find that community resilience may help to mitigate the negative impact of oppression and improve outcomes for LGBTQ people of color; however, LGBTQ people of color may also experience increased minority stress and rejection due to holding multiple marginalized identity statuses (Parmenter et al., 2021). In cognitive science, Belem and colleagues (2021) examine how the combination of intersectionality and resilience theory may provide a more holistic approach to understanding the experiences of individuals who are bilingual. They highlight that for individuals who are bilingual (predominantly people of color), their experiences exist within different cultural, individual, and societal contexts that are important to consider. Lastly, in psychological research, Vance and colleagues propose that suicide-related behavior and outcomes in Black women cannot be studied if not from an intersectional perspective. Within their research, they demonstrate gendered racial experiences that impact suicide risk and resilience for Black women (Vance et al., 2023). Collectively, these studies highlight that it is imperative to examine the relationship between resilience and health outcomes from an intersectional perspective. Especially because many Black Americans lie at multiple different intersections of identity, oppression, and power. Additionally, intersectional studies and frameworks rarely give attention to overlapping strengths-based resilience processes or wellness and health-promoting resources (Hankivsky, 2012). By informing resilience research through an intersectional lens, there is an opportunity not only to better expose multiple layers of inequity and disadvantage occurring from intersecting forms of oppression, but also to encourage the inclusion of complex, strengths-based factors of individual and social resilience.

8.5 Conclusion and Future Directions

Wellness and resilience are interconnected and necessary for the continual survival of Black people. A culturally specific redefinition of resilience shifts the focus from the ability to overcome to the ability to recover. The redefinition of resilience is grounded in a Black psychology perspective, which emphasizes the interdependent connection between the mind, body, and spirit (Phillips, 1990; Tsa-Tsala, 1997). When thinking about resilience, it is more than just the physical body overcoming a challenge it is also the ways in which one's mental health and spiritual well-being are simultaneously impacted by difficult circumstances. Taking a holistic approach to understanding resilience enables the ability to rethink intervention strategies to better support the well-being and overall existence of Black people. This chapter attempts to provide a holistic intervention framework by offering a theoretical model that acknowledges intersecting forms of oppression while highlighting strength-based factors that can support Black people's resilience. The proposed theoretical model takes an intersectional and strengths-based approach to understanding resilience among Black people within the context of the socio-ecological model. The model allows for systematic facilitation of intervention and prevention strategies to mitigate harm from oppression and increase resilience.

Questions for Thought and Discussion

1. What is the relationship between racial identity and psychological well-being for Black individuals? How does the endorsement of high levels of racial identity serve as a protective factor?
2. How do you view your racial identity (negatively and positively), and what impact has that had on your well-being?
3. How do intersectional identities predispose or protect an individual against adverse outcomes?
4. What strategies do you currently use, or might you begin to use to help nurture your inner resiliency and strengths?
5. How do culturally specific ways of coping such as Africultural coping techniques, contribute to the psychological well-being and resilience of Black individuals?
6. How can research and interventions in psychology and public health promote resilience and well-being in Black individuals?

Conflict of Interest We have no known conflict of interest to disclose

References

Alang, S. M. (2019). Mental health care among blacks in America: Confronting racism and constructing solutions. *Health Services Research, 54*(2), 346–355. https://doi.org/10.1111/1475-6773.13115

Arnold, L. M., Crofford, L. J., Martin, S. A., Young, J. P., & Sharma, U. (2007). The effect of anxiety and depression on improvements in pain in a randomized, controlled trial of pregabalin for treatment of fibromyalgia. *Pain Medicine, 8*(8), 633–638. https://doi.org/10.1111/j.1526-4637.2007.00332.x

Banks, K. H., & Kohn-Wood, L. P. (2007). The influence of racial identity profiles on the relationship between racial discrimination and depressive symptoms. *Journal of Black Psychology, 33*(3), 331–354. https://doi.org/10.1177/0095798407302540

Belgrave, F. Z., & Allison, K. W. (2014). Psychosocial adaptation and mental health. In *African American psychology: From Africa to America* (3rd ed., pp. 409–444). Sage.

Boyd, D. T., Jones, K. V., Quinn, C. R., Gale, A., Williams, E. D. G., & Lateef, H. (2022). The mental health of black youth affected by community violence: Family and school context as pathways to resilience. *Children, 9*(2), 259. https://doi.org/10.3390/children9020259

Bronfenbrenner, U. (1979). Contexts of child rearing: Problems and prospects. *American Psychologist, 34*(10), 844–850. https://doi.org/10.1037/0003-066X.34.10.844

Bronfenbrenner, U. (1988). Interacting systems in human development: Research paradigms: Present and future. In *Persons in context: Developmental processes* (pp. 25–49). Cambridge University Press. https://doi.org/10.1017/cbo9780511663949.003

Buttram, M. E. (2019). The social environmental context of resilience among substance-using African American/black men who have sex with men. *Journal of Homosexuality, 67*(6), 816–832. https://doi.org/10.1080/00918369.2018.1557952

Carroll, K. K. (2010). A genealogical review of the worldview framework in African-centered psychology. *The Journal of Pan African Studies, 3*(8).

Case, K. (2013). *Deconstructing privilege*. Routledge. https://doi.org/10.4324/9780203081877

Catabay, C. J., Stockman, J. K., Campbell, J. C., & Tsuyuki, K. (2019). Perceived stress and mental health: The mediating roles of social support and resilience among black women exposed to sexual violence. *Journal of Affective Disorders, 259*, 143–149. https://doi.org/10.1016/j.jad.2019.08.037

Cho, S., Crenshaw, K. W., & McCall, L. (2013). Toward a field of intersectionality studies: Theory, applications, and praxis. *Signs: Journal of Women in Culture and Society, 38*(4), 785–810. https://doi.org/10.1086/669608

Cokley, K., Palmer, B., & Stone, S. (2019). Toward a black (and diverse) psychology: The scholarly legacy of Joseph White. *Journal of Black Psychology, 45*(2), 112–121.

Cole, E. R. (2009). Intersectionality and research in psychology. *American Psychologist, 64*(3), 170–180. https://doi.org/10.1037/a0014564

Collective, C. R. (1983). The Combahee river collective statement. *Home Girls: A Black Feminist Anthology, 1*, 264–274.

Collins, P. H. (1986). Learning from the outsider within: The socioecological significance of black feminist thought. *Social Problems, 33*(6), 14–32. https://doi.org/10.2307/800672

Constantine, M. G., Donnelly, P. C., & Myers, L. J. (2002). Collective self-esteem and Africultural coping styles in African American adolescents. *Journal of Black Studies, 32*(6), 698–710. https://doi.org/10.1177/00234702032006004

Cousins, N. (1989). *Head first: The biology of hope* (1st ed.). Dutton.

Crenshaw, K. (1989). Demarginalizing the intersection of race and sex: A black feminist critique of antidiscrimination doctrine, feminist theory and antiracist politics. *u. Chi. Legal f.*, 139.

Curry, M., Lipscomb, A., Ashley, W., & McCarty-Caplan, D. (2022). Black barbershops: Exploring informal mental health settings within the community. *Journal of Humanities and Social Sciences Studies, 4*(1), 60–69. https://doi.org/10.32996/jhsss.2022.4.1.6

Do, D. P., Locklar, L. R., & Florsheim, P. (2019). Triple jeopardy: The joint impact of racial segregation and neighborhood poverty on the mental health of black Americans. *Social Psychiatry and Psychiatric Epidemiology, 54*(5), 533–541. https://doi.org/10.1007/s00127-019-01654-5

Fergus, S., & Zimmerman, M. A. (2005). Adolescent resilience: A framework for understanding healthy development in the face of risk. *Annual Review of Public Health, 26*, 399–419. https://doi.org/10.1146/annurev.publhealth.26.021304.144357

Follins, L. D., Garrett-Walker, J. J., & Lewis, M. K. (2014). Resilience in black lesbian, gay, bisexual, and transgender individuals: A critical review of the literature. *Journal of Gay & Lesbian Mental Health, 18*(2), 190–212. https://doi.org/10.1080/19359705.2013.828343

Gaston, M. H., Porter, G. K., & Thomas, V. G. (2007). Prime time sister circles: Evaluating a gender-specific, culturally relevant health intervention to decrease major risk factors in mid-life African-American women. *Journal of the National Medical Association, 99*(4), 428–438. https://doi.org/10.1016/j.jnma.2015.12.001

Gibson, S. M., Bouldin, B. M., Stokes, M. N., Lozada, F. T., & Hope, E. C. (2022). Cultural racism and depression in black adolescents: Examining racial socialization and racial identity as moderators. *Journal of Research on Adolescence, 32*(1), 41–48. https://doi.org/10.1111/jora.12698

Goldstein, S., & Brooks, R. B. (2013). Why study resilience? In S. Goldstein & R. Brooks (Eds.), *Handbook of resilience in children* (pp. 3–14). Springer. https://doi.org/10.1007/978-1-4614-3661-4_1

Gonzalez, J. S., Safren, S. A., Delahanty, L. M., Cagliero, E., Wexler, D. J., Meigs, J. B., & Grant, R. W. (2008). Symptoms of depression prospectively predict poorer self-care in patients with type 2 diabetes. *Diabetic Medicine, 25*(9), 1102–1107. https://doi.org/10.1111/j.1464-5491.2008.02535.x

Hadden, S. E. (2003). *Slave patrols: Law and violence in Virginia and the Carolinas*. Harvard University Press. https://doi.org/10.2307/1350169

Hampton-Anderson, J. N., Watson-Singleton, N. N., Mekawi, Y., Dunn, S. E., & Kaslow, N. J. (2022). Intimate partner violence, existential well-being, and Africultural coping in African American women. *Journal of Aggression, Maltreatment & Trauma, 31*(5), 660–676. https://doi.org/10.1080/10926771.2022.2038751

Hankivsky, O. (2012). Women's health, men's health, and gender and health: Implications of intersectionality. *Social Science & Medicine, 74*(11), 1712–1720. https://doi.org/10.1016/j.socscimed.2011.11.029

Hankivsky, O., Grace, D., Hunting, G., Giesbrecht, M., Fridkin, A., Rudrum, S., et al. (2014). An intersectionality-based policy analysis framework: Critical reflections on a methodology for advancing equity. *International Journal for Equity in Health, 13*(1), 1–16. https://doi.org/10.1186/s12939-014-0119-x

Hartman, S. (2008). *Lose your mother: A journey along the Atlantic slave route*. Macmillan. https://doi.org/10.1017/S0021875810000071

Hawkins, D. S. (2022). "After Philando, I had to take a sick day to recover": Psychological distress, trauma and police brutality in the black community. *Health Communication, 37*(9), 1113–1122. https://doi.org/10.1037/vio0000438

Hine, D. C. (2007). *Ar'n't I a woman?: Female slaves in the plantation south*: Twenty years after. *The Journal of African American History, 92*(1), 13–21.

James Myers, L., Lodge, T., Speight, S. L., & Haggins, K. (2022). The necessity of an emic paradigm in psychology. *Journal of Humanistic Psychology, 62*(4), 488–515. https://doi.org/10.1177/00221678211048568

Jones, H. L., Cross, W. E., Jr., & DeFour, D. C. (2007). Race-related stress, racial identity attitudes, and mental health among black women. *Journal of Black Psychology, 33*(2), 208–231. https://doi.org/10.1177/0095798407299517

Kambon, K. K. (2012). *African/black psychology in the American context: An African-centered approach*. Nubian Nation Publications.

Kilanowski, J. F. (2017). Breadth of the socio-ecological model. *Journal of Agromedicine, 22*(4), 295–297. https://doi.org/10.1080/1059924X.2017.1358971

Kim, J. H., Islam, S. J., Topel, M. L., Ko, Y. A., Mujahid, M. S., Vaccarino, V., et al. (2020). Individual psychosocial resilience, neighborhood context, and cardiovascular health in black adults: A multilevel investigation from the Morehouse-Emory Cardiovascular Center for Health Equity Study. *Circulation: Cardiovascular Quality and Outcomes, 13*(10), e006638. https://doi.org/10.1161/CIRCOUTCOMES.120.006638

Krause, N., Emmons, R. A., Ironson, G., & Hill, P. C. (2017). General feelings of gratitude, gratitude to god, and hemoglobin A1c: Exploring variations by gender. *The Journal of Positive Psychology, 12*(6), 639–650. https://doi.org/10.1080/17439760.2017.1326520

Lateef, H., Amoako, E. O., Nartey, P., Tan, J., & Joe, S. (2022). Black youth and African-centered interventions: A systematic review. *Research on Social Work Practice, 32*(1), 3–12. https://doi.org/10.1177/10497315211003322

LaVeist, T. A., Gaskin, D., & Richard, P. (2011). Estimating the economic burden of racial health inequalities in the United States. *International Journal of Health Services, 41*(2), 231–238. https://doi.org/10.2190/HS.41.2.c

Legler, S. R., Beale, E. E., Celano, C. M., Beach, S. R., & Healy, B. C. (2019). State gratitude for one's life and health after an acute coronary syndrome: Prospective associations with physical activity medical adherence and re-hospitalizations. *The Journal of Positive Psychology, 14*(3), 283–291. https://doi.org/10.1080/17439760.2017.1414295

le Roux, S., Denton, R. A., Malan, L., & Malan, N. T. (2022). Coping with chronic stress during COVID-19 and beyond–a faith perspective. *die Skriflig/In Luce Verbi, 56*(1), 11. https://doi.org/10.4102/ids.v56i1.2823

Lewis-Coles, M. A. E. L., & Constantine, M. G. (2006). Racism-related stress, Africultural coping, and religious problem-solving among African Americans. *Cultural Diversity and Ethnic Minority Psychology, 12*(3), 433. https://doi.org/10.1037/1099-9809.12.3.433

Lydiard, R. B. (2001). Irritable bowel syndrome, anxiety, and depression: What are the links? *Journal of Clinical Psychiatry, 62*, 38–47.

Massie, M. J. (2004). Prevalence of depression in patients with cancer. *JNCI Monographs, 2004*(32), 57–71. https://doi.org/10.1093/jncimonographs/lgh014

Mbilishaka, A. M. (2018a). Strands of intimacy: Black Women's narratives of hair and intimate relationships with men. *Journal of Black Sexuality and Relationships, 5*(1), 43–61. https://doi.org/10.1353/bsr.2018.0014

Mbilishaka, A. M. (2018b). Black lives (and stories) matter: Race narrative therapy in black hair care spaces. *Community Psychology in Global Perspective, 4*(2), 22–33. https://doi.org/10.1285/i24212113v4i2p22

Mbilishaka, A. M., Mbande, A., Gulley, C. & Mbande, T. (2021). Faded fresh tapers and line-ups: Centering barbershop hair stories in understanding gendered racial socialization for black men. *Psychology of Men & Masculinities, 22*(1), 166–176. https://doi.org/10.1037/men0000317

McDonough, I. M., Byrd, D. R., & Choi, S. L. (2022). Resilience resources may buffer some middle aged and older black Americans from memory decline despite experiencing discrimination. *Social Science & Medicine, 316*, 114998. https://doi.org/10.1016/j.socscimed.2022.114998

Miller-Matero, L. R., Saulino, C., Clark, S., Bugenski, M., Eshelman, A., & Eisenstein, D. (2016). When treating the pain is not enough: A multidisciplinary approach for chronic pelvic pain. *Archives Women's Mental Health, 19*(2), 349–354. https://doi.org/10.1007/s00737-015-0537-9

Morrison, K. S., & Hopkins, R. (2019). Cultural identity, Africultural coping strategies, and depression as predictors of suicidal ideations and attempts among African American female college students. *Journal of Black Psychology, 45*(1), 3–25. https://doi.org/10.1177/0095798418813511

Murry, V. M., Gonzalez, C. M., Hanebutt, R. A., Bulgin, D., Coates, E. E., Inniss-Thompson, M. N., Debreaux, M. L., Wilson, W. E., Abel, D., & Cortez, M. B. (2022). Longitudinal study of the cascading effects of racial discrimination on parenting and adjustment among African American youth. *Attachment & Human Development, 24*(3), 322–338. https://doi.org/10.1080/14616734.2021.1976926

Neal-Barnett, A., Stadulis, R., Murray, M., Payne, M. R., Thomas, A., & Salley, B. B. (2011). Sister circles as a culturally relevant intervention for anxious black women. *Clinical Psychology: Science and Practice, 18*(3), 266–273. https://doi.org/10.1111/j.1468-2850.2011.01258.x

Neblett, E. W., Jr. (2019). Racism and health: Challenges and future directions in behavioral and psychological research. *Cultural Diversity and Ethnic Minority Psychology, 25*(1), 12.

Ojelade, I. I., McCray, K., Meyers, J., & Ashby, J. (2014). Use of indigenous African healing practices as a mental health intervention. *Journal of Black Psychology, 40*(6), 491–519. https://doi.org/10.1177/0095798414533345

Parmenter, J. G., Galliher, R. V., Wong, E., & Perez, D. (2021). An intersectional approach to understanding LGBTQ+ people of color's access to LGBTQ+ community resilience. *Journal of Counseling Psychology, 68*, 629. https://doi.org/10.1037/cou0000578

Phillips, F. B. (1990). NTU psychotherapy: An Afrocentric approach. *Journal of Black Psychology, 17*(1), 55–74. https://doi.org/10.1177/00957984900171005

Prince, M., Patel, V., Saxena, S., Maj, M., Maselko, J., Phillips, M. R., & Rahman, A. (2007). No health without mental health. *The Lancet, 370*(9590), 859–877. https://doi.org/10.1016/S0140-6736(07)61238-0

Pyant, C. T., & Yanico, B. J. (1991). Relationship of racial identity and gender-role attitudes to black women's psychological well-being. *Journal of Counseling Psychology, 38*(3), 315. https://doi.org/10.1037/0022-0167.38.3.315

Rowley, S. J., Sellers, R. M., Chavous, T. M., & Smith, M. A. (1998). The relationship between racial identity and self-esteem in African American college and high school students. *Journal of Personality and Social Psychology, 74*(3), 715. https://doi.org/10.1037/0022-3514.74.3.715

Scioli, A., Scioli-Salter, E. R., Sykes, K., Anderson, C., & Fedele, M. (2016). The positive contributions of hope to maintaining and restoring health: An integrative, mixed-method approach. *The Journal of Positive Psychology, 11*(2), 135–148. https://doi.org/10.1080/17439760.2015.1037858

Seligman, M. E. (2002). Positive psychology, positive prevention, and positive therapy. *Handbook of Positive Psychology, 2*(2002), 3–12.

Sellers, R. M., Copeland-Linder, N., Martin, P. P., & Lewis, R. L. H. (2006). Racial identity matters: The relationship between racial discrimination and psychological functioning in African American adolescents. *Journal of Research on Adolescence, 16*(2), 187–216. https://doi.org/10.1111/j.1532-7795.2006.00128.x

Shaw, J., McLean, K. C., Taylor, B., Swartout, K., & Querna, K. (2016). Beyond resilience: Why we need to look at systems too. *Psychology of Violence, 6*(1), 34. https://doi.org/10.1037/vio0000020

Snyder, C. R. (2004). Hope and depression: A light in the darkness. *Journal of Social and Clinical Psychology, 23*(3), 347. https://doi.org/10.1521/jscp.23.3.347.35458

Staggers-Hakim, R. (2016). The nation's unprotected children and the ghost of Mike Brown, or the impact of national police killings on the health and social development of African American boys. *Journal of Human Behavior in the Social Environment, 26*(3–4), 390–399. https://doi.org/10.1080/10911359.2015.1132864

Stern, J. A., Barbarin, O., & Cassidy, J. (2022). Working toward anti-racist perspectives in attachment theory, research, and practice. *Attachment & Human Development, 24*(3), 392–422. https://doi.org/10.1080/14616734.2021.1976933

Tsala-Tsala, J. (1997). Beliefs and disease in Cameroon. In S. N. Madu, P. K. Baguma, & A. Pritz (Eds.), *Psychotherapy in Africa: First investigation* (p. 44). World Council for Psychotherapy.

Tynes, B. M., Willis, H. A., Stewart, A. M., & Hamilton, M. W. (2019). Race-related traumatic events online and mental health among adolescents of color. *Journal of Adolescent Health, 65*(3), 371–377. https://doi.org/10.1016/j.jadohealth.2019.03.006

Utsey, S. O., Adams, E. P., & Bolden, M. (2000). Development and initial validation of the Agricultural coping systems inventory. *Journal of Black Psychology, 26*(2), 194–215. https://doi.org/10.1177/0095798400026002005

Utsey, S. O., Bolden, M. A., Lanier, Y., & Williams, O., III. (2007). Examining the role of culture-specific coping as a predictor of resilient outcomes in African Americans from high-risk urban communities. *Journal of Black Psychology, 33*(1), 75–93. https://doi.org/10.1177/0095798406295094

Vance, M. M., Wade, J. M., Brandy, M., & Webster, A. R. (2023). Contextualizing black women's mental health in the twenty-first century: Gendered racism and suicide-related behavior. *Journal of Racial and Ethnic Health Disparities, 10*, 83–92. https://doi.org/10.1007/s40615-021-01198-y

Vandiver, B. J. (2020). Message from the editor-in-chief: Racism as public health crisis. *Journal of Black Psychology, 46*(5), 347–350. https://doi.org/10.1177/0095798420956806

Victor, R. G., Ravenell, J. E., Freeman, A., Leonard, D., Bhat, D. G., Shafiq, M., et al. (2011). Effectiveness of a barber-based intervention for improving hypertension control in black men: The BARBER-1 study: A cluster randomized trial. *Archives of Internal Medicine, 171*(4), 342–350. https://doi.org/10.1001/archinternmed.2010.390

Warner, L. R., & Shields, S. A. (2013). The intersections of sexuality, gender, and race: Identity research at the crossroads. *Sex Roles, 68*(11), 803–810. https://doi.org/10.1007/s11199-013-0281-4

Watson-Thompson, J., Hassaballa, R. H., Valentini, S. H., Schultz, J. A., Vanchy Kadavasal, P., Harsin, J. D., Thompson, V. M., Hassaballa, I. H., Esiaka, C. C., & Thompson, E. C. (2022). Actively addressing systemic racism using a behavioral community approach. *Behavior and Social Issues, 31*, 297–326. https://doi.org/10.1007/s42822-022-00101-6

White, J. (1970). Toward a black psychology. *Ebony, 25*(11), 44–45.

Wilson, S. L., Sellers, S., Solomon, C., & Holsey-Hyman, M. (2017). Exploring the link between black racial identity and mental health. *Journal of Depression and Anxiety, 6*(3), 1–4. https://doi.org/10.4172/2167-1044.1000272

Yip, T., Seaton, E. K., & Sellers, R. M. (2006). African American racial identity across the lifespan: Identity status, identity content, and depressive symptoms. *Child Development, 77*(5), 1504–1517. https://doi.org/10.1111/j.1467-8624.2006.00950.x

Index

J. M. Koch et al. (eds.), *Identity as Resilience in Minoritized Communities*, Emerging Issues in Family and Individual Resilience,
https://doi.org/10.1007/978-3-031-38977-1

9783031389764